THE 5-MINUTE
OSTEOPATHIC
MANIPULATIVE
MEDICINE CONSULT

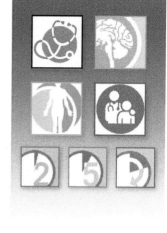

THE 5-MINUTE
OSTEOPATHIC
MANIPULATIVE
MEDICINE CONSULT

SECOND EDITION

Millicent King Channell, DO, MA, FAAO
Assistant Dean for Curriculum
Professor, Department of Osteopathic Manipulative Medicine
Rowan University, School of Osteopathic Medicine
Stratford, New Jersey

David C. Mason, DO, MBA, FACOFP
ONMM and FM/ONMM Residency Director Medical City
    Fort Worth
Interim Senior Associate Dean of Academic Affairs
Associate Professor Department of Family Medicine and
    Osteopathic Manipulative Medicine
UNTHSC—Texas College of Osteopathic Medicine
Fort Worth, Texas

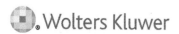 Wolters Kluwer

Philadelphia • Baltimore • New York • London
Buenos Aires • Hong Kong • Sydney • Tokyo

Acquisitions Editor: Matt Hauber
Development Editor: Amy Millholen
Editorial Coordinator: John Larkin
Marketing Manager: Phyllis Hitner
Production Project Manager: Bridgett Dougherty
Design Coordinator: Holly McLaughlin
Manufacturing Coordinator: Margie Orzech-Zeranko
Prepress Vendor: Absolute Service, Inc.

Second Edition

Library of Congress Cataloging-in-Publication Data

Names: Channell, Millicent King, author. | Mason, David C., DO, author.
Title: The 5-minute osteopathic manipulative medicine consult / Millicent
 King Channell, David C. Mason.
Other titles: Five-minute osteopathic manipulative medicine consult |
 5-minute consult (Series)
Description: Second edition. | Philadelphia : Wolters Kluwer, [2020] |
 Series: 5-minute consult series | Includes bibliographical references and
 index.
Identifiers: LCCN 2019005288 | ISBN 9781496396501 (paperback)
Subjects: | MESH: Manipulation, Osteopathic--methods | Handbook
Classification: LCC RZ342.9 | NLM WB 39 | DDC 615.5/33--dc23 LC record
available at https://lccn.loc.gov/2019005288

CD062024

DEDICATION

*To family, friends, and colleagues who continue
to support us in all the projects to promote the
profession we love so much.*

*To all those in search of health, we hope this helps
your journey.*

PREFACE

Incorporating osteopathic manipulative medicine (OMM) into the modern 7-minute office visit is not easy. The goal of this book is to give practitioners who are not osteopathic specialists some direction in where to begin and focus their attention, given a particular disease process and the time constraints of today's medical practices. Each patient should be individually evaluated and an appropriate treatment plan devised given the patient's history and physical exam.

This book is not intended to be a comprehensive collection of techniques; there are several excellent books in publication to provide that service. This book is also not intended to create a "cookbook approach" to OMM. That is worth repeating: *This book is not intended as a cookbook of OMM*. Using palpatory skills and an osteopathic exam to properly diagnose somatic dysfunction is the best guide to the appropriate application of osteopathic manipulation. However, osteopathic students and physicians have all been trained to do evaluations and treatments of the entire body that last 30 to 60 minutes. Many osteopathic students and physicians have difficulty focusing osteopathic treatments to the presenting problem, and therefore do not do it at all.

Limited time is one of the main reasons OMM is often overlooked. Therefore, special attention is placed on outlining time-efficient treatment plans. Physicians can then decide how much time they have for a particular office visit and treat patients with techniques that should be efficacious. This approach may also facilitate revisits, for which more complete osteopathic treatment can be planned and sufficient time scheduled. It is anticipated that this resource will help students and physicians use techniques under such time constraints. The listing of areas of potential somatic dysfunction and suggested treatments should facilitate the application of osteopathic manipulation in clinical scenarios that are otherwise familiar to the reader. Therefore, proper medical evaluation and treatment are not included in this text; other 5-Minute clinical consult books may be used for that purpose. This book is intended to add osteopathic manipulative treatment (OMT) adjunctively to the standard medical treatment of the diagnoses discussed.

Physicians are very good at devising a list of differential diagnoses and a treatment plan based on the diagnosis. Somatic dysfunctions are commonly overlooked on the differential list, and adding OMT to the treatment plan is therefore neglected. These are missed opportunities to immediately help our patients, highlight our osteopathic distinctiveness, and appropriately code and bill for an additional office procedure. This text continually reminds the user of proper diagnosis, documentation, coding, and billing.

PREFACE

It is our objective to put osteopathic manipulation into the hands of all physicians, not just OMM specialists. We hope this book helps to bridge the gap for those students and physicians who need a little direction on how to formulate focused OMM treatment plans.

MILLICENT KING CHANNELL, DO, MA, FAAO

DAVID C. MASON, DO, MBA, FACOFP

ACKNOWLEDGMENTS

Special thanks to several individuals who have helped us complete this project. Thank you Karen T. Snider, DO, FAAO, FNAOME, for her contributions to our literature searches. Our gratitude goes to our photographic models: Desean Lee, OMS2; Cara Pietrolungo, OMS2; Trinava Roy, OMS2; Brittany Snow, OMS2; and Ashton Whaley. Thank you to our illustrator, Bob McBride, who delivered superb artwork making some difficult concepts easy to visualize. And to our photographers, Steve Seidler and Miral Vaghasia, DO, whose pictures are beautifully done. We would also like to offer our appreciation to our mentors and colleagues for their wisdom and guidance. Most importantly, we would like to thank our families for their sacrifices and support of this and all of our professional endeavors. Our families mean more to us than words here can convey.

THE IMPORTANCE OF THIS BOOK

Originally born out of a desire to bridge a gap in application of acquired knowledge, this book has many uses during and postosteopathic medical training. Both authors graduated from osteopathic medical schools and completed osteopathic family medicine residencies only to realize there was no clear education of how and when to use osteopathic manipulative treatment in practice. Integrating osteopathic principles and manipulative practice requires diagnosis of somatic dysfunction and skilled application of technique to resolve those somatic dysfunctions. Osteopathic medical schools provide a strong didactic and laboratory foundation with an average of 200 hours dedicated to training in the first 2 preclinical years. These curricula take many forms and organizational schema. Not all provide opportunities to practice these skills in a clinical setting with direct mentored supervision prior to graduation. Lack of mentoring and guided practice during clinical education often leads to omission of osteopathic diagnosis and treatment in the patient encounter throughout the rest of training and into practice.

Several changes have occurred since the first edition of *The 5-Minute Osteopathic Manipulative Medicine Consult*, which make it even more relevant today. Some schools have updated curricula with improved integration of osteopathic concepts and application of technique and need resources to reinforce these concepts. The Comprehensive Osteopathic Medical Licensing Examination of the United States Level 2-Performance Evaluation (COMLEX Level 2-PE) standardized exam has also helped place an emphasis on the need to integrate osteopathic thinking and diagnostic and treatment technique skills. Unification of graduate medical education through the Accreditation Council for Graduate Medical Education (ACGME) is well underway and due to be completed in 2020. These changes provide even more opportunities to highlight the distinctiveness of osteopathic training and practice. Osteopathic recognition is a distinction for residencies who integrate osteopathic principles, practice, and research into their training.

WHO SHOULD USE THIS REFERENCE?

FIRST- AND SECOND-YEAR MEDICAL STUDENTS

Whether you are attending an osteopathic medical school that has a presentation-based curriculum, a systems-based curriculum, or another organization of medical knowledge, this book can help you make a link between the basic sciences, medical diagnoses, and the osteopathic principles and application of technique in a clear and quick manner. It is meant for efficient review and putting the full picture together. This is a good supplement to your school's required manuals and references to learn and demonstrate competency of osteopathic medicine.

THE IMPORTANCE OF THIS BOOK

THIRD- AND FOURTH-YEAR MEDICAL STUDENTS

Armed with diagnostic skills to find somatic dysfunction and ready to apply several techniques to each body region, there is still a gap on how and when to apply these skills. "Why would I look in these body regions when someone presents with cough?" or "I have already diagnosed the patient with asthma?" This text facilitates your thought process to incorporate osteopathic principles using your knowledge of anatomy and physiology to rationally guide you through a focused osteopathic exam.

RESIDENTS IN TRAINING AND THEIR PROGRAMS

Osteopathic recognition is a new distinction provided by the ACGME to programs that apply and meet standards of training and research in osteopathic medicine. To the faculty and residents of these programs, this book can provide a guide for integration into clinical practice as well as didactic sessions on the medical topics discussed. Many residency directors have provided positive feedback which has been incorporated into this second edition, in order to help programs reach their educational goals

Additionally, repetitious discussion of appropriate documentation, coding, and billing practices are provided here to meet medical practice competencies and assure appropriate use of somatic dysfunction ICD-10 codes and osteopathic manipulative treatment CPT codes.

PHYSICIANS IN PRACTICE

Many physicians already in practice wish a refresher in a time-efficient way to incorporate osteopathic manipulative principles and treatment in order to better serve their patients and provide a more comprehensive medical experience for them. Adjunctive treatments are sought by our patients wishing to minimize pharmaceuticals and surgical interventions until more conservative approaches have been exhausted. This guide reminds the physician of the connections of anatomy and physiology to their patient's medical conditions. It reminds us of our basic osteopathic training and the ease of incorporating diagnosis and treatment even into the busiest practices. Discussion and reminders of appropriate documentation, coding, and billing provides the fundamentals to be reimbursed for the valuable treatment being provided for our patients.

ORGANIZATION OF DIAGNOSIS CHAPTERS

THE BASICS

A quick description of the diagnosis is provided. It can be used as an easy-to-understand explanation for patients in order to start a conversation about their condition and how you think osteopathic principles can help you better treat them.

Physiology and associated somatic dysfunction is a reference to the autonomic nervous system and other pertinent anatomy related to the condition. The areas of parasympathetic and sympathetic innervation are reviewed in order to guide your investigation into likely areas of somatic dysfunction. Lymphatic and biomechanically relevant areas of anatomy are added next. These areas of the patient should be high-yield areas for somatic dysfunction. Every patient is unique and may have additional areas of related somatic dysfunction and/or may not have associated somatic dysfunction in these regions at this time. This should help focus your exam to most likely areas of somatic dysfunction to help you become more efficient in rationally considering how somatic dysfunction can be a primary or a secondary contributor to your patient's overall health and disease related to the topic.

TREATMENT

Treatment offers suggestions to get you started with OMT to some of the most relevant area where you have now identified somatic dysfunction. These are certainly not the only techniques that may be useful; time and practice will help you become proficient with choosing an appropriate treatment modality for the patient in front of you. You may have more proficiency or comfort with certain treatment models and are encouraged to use what you feel is most appropriate for your patient.

2-MINUTE, 5-MINUTE, EXTENDED TREATMENT

Time is a factor in medical practice. If there is very limited time to treat the patient at this visit, start with the suggested treatment techniques and areas of treatment under the 2-Minute Treatment. If you have more time, proceed to the 5-Minute Treatment and, if possible, the Extended Treatment suggestions applying any of the techniques to the areas of somatic dysfunction you found on your focused examination of the patient. Skip any areas where you did not identify somatic dysfunction and consider bringing your patient back for a reevaluation of their medical complaint/diagnosis and reexamine them for the presence of somatic dysfunction at that return visit.

BILLING AND CODING

ICD-10 CODES

There are 10 ICD-10 codes used for somatic dysfunctions. They are M99.00 Head SD, M99.01 Cervical SD, M99.02 Thoracic SD, M99.03 Lumbar SD, M99.04 Sacrum SD, M99.05 Pelvic SD, M99.06 Lower Extremity SD, M99.07 Upper Extremity SD, M99.08 Rib SD, and M99.09 Abdomen and Other SD.

SOMATIC DYSFUNCTION

Somatic dysfunction is defined as the impaired or altered function of related components of the somatic system including the skeletal, arthrodial, and myofascial structures and their related vascular, lymphatic, and neural elements. The basic physical findings associated with somatic dysfunction are (T) tissue texture changes, (A) asymmetry on static exam, (R) range of motion deficits, and (T) tenderness. These TART components can and should be used when documenting somatic dysfunctions in your patient charts. Further positional diagnoses related to Fryette's rules in the thoracic and lumbar spine, cardinal motions available to the cervical spine and standard cardinal positions of motion for pelvic, sacrum, extremities, and ribs may be used to further define somatic dysfunction. Certain nomenclature is more helpful for certain treatment models than others such as tenderpoints related to strain counterstrain or fascial planes of motion restriction/bind or ease for myofascial release techniques.

Once somatic dysfunction is identified, a region and the appropriate ICD-10 codes should be assigned. This is the only indication for using osteopathic manipulative treatment and should be linked to the use of the OMT procedure codes in the following text.

E&M CPT CODES

Evaluation and management (E&M) codes reflect mainly the cognitive and physical exam of a patient encounter. There are graduated sets of codes based on place of service and new or established visits. Refer to appropriate references to become familiar with all of the guidelines in order to choose the most appropriate code for the patient encounter you are documenting. The following bullets are important to consider:

- New visit codes (99201 to 99205) require all three components be considered: history, physical exam, and medical decision making.
- Established visit codes (99211 to 99215) only require you consider two of three components: history, physical exam, and medical decision making.
- Hospital codes (99221 to 99223, 99231 to 99232, 99238 to 99239) and long-term care codes (99304 to 99310) may also be combined with OMT procedure codes using the .25 modifier when appropriate.

OMT PROCEDURE CODES

There are five OMT procedure codes 98925 to 98929. They are based on the number of body regions treated with OMT. Upper or lower extremity each only counts as one even if both right and left sides are treated; this is also true for ribs if right and left are treated. Each region should only be counted once per visit even if multiple somatic dysfunctions or segments are treated in the same area on the same day.

OMT CPT CODES	
1–2 regions	98925
3–4 regions	98926
5–6 regions	98927
7–8 regions	98928
9–10 regions	98929

OMT is a procedure and should be documented in a procedure note, which should include all of the elements of a procedure note. This should include physical findings and the resultant somatic dysfunction diagnosis, the patient's verbal consent, the osteopathic manipulative treatment performed, and the patient's response to treatment.

MODIFIER 25

Modifier 25 is added to the E&M code to signify that on the same day, as an E&M code was performed, a separately identifiable procedure was done. In this case, the procedure is OMT, but it is the same modifier that is used if an injection or other office procedure is performed.

DOCUMENT YOUR HISTORY, EXAM, AND DECISION MAKING

Osteopathic manipulative treatment is not an intervention meant to be done in isolation and as such should not be prescribed in multiple sessions without thorough reevaluation of the patient's presentation, history, physical exam, and review of the physician's medical decision making. Patients should not be told to come back specifically for OMT because it may not be indicated at the next visit. Only if a history and physical exam rule in and out other causes of the presenting symptoms and define that somatic dysfunction is present, either as the underlying (primary) cause of the presentation or in conjunction (secondary) to another medical issue related to the presentation should OMT be used. OMT should only be implemented after the physician reasons that it is safe to perform, has selected an appropriate technique that is expected to reduce or remove the somatic dysfunction, and improves the related presentation.

Additionally, in the medical decision making, the physician should review any medical management, consider alternatives to treatment, and decide if further radiological or laboratory workup is needed and if additional resources such as referrals, exercise, nutrition, or other therapies would be beneficial at this time. All of these should be documented as any competent physician should be doing as part of their E&M services and as this is unrelated to the pre- and postapplication of OMT. Physicians who then determine it is appropriately indicated and safe to proceed with OMT are to use the OMT procedure codes and append a 25 modifier to the E&M code.

ICD-10 CODES FOR SOMATIC DYSFUNCTION

Region	ICD-10
Head	M99.00
Cervical	M99.01
Thoracic	M99.02
Lumbar	M99.03
Sacrum	M99.04
Pelvic	M99.05
Lower Extremity	M99.06
Upper Extremity	M99.07
Ribs	M99.08
Abdomen and Other	M99.09

OMM PRECEPTING GUIDE

OMM PRECEPTING GUIDE

Technique	Direct/ Indirect	Active/ Passive	Mechanism of Action
Soft tissue	Direct	Passive	A technique that usually involves kneading, stretching, deep pressure, inhibition, and/or traction while monitoring tissue response and motion changes by palpation. This technique is a form of myofascial treatment.
MFR	Direct or indirect	Passive	A technique that engages the fascia of the tissues and by using thermodynamic and mechanotransduction from the physician's hands to the patient's soft tissue and fascia; can cause piezoelectric changes which can soften, elongate, relax, and release restricted fascial tissues
Lymphatic	Direct	Passive	Mechanical compression via physician's force leads to mobilization of lymphatic fluid.
CS	Indirect	Passive	A technique where a tenderpoint of a dysfunctional muscle or joint is put into its position of greatest comfort in order to reduce the continuing inappropriate, hypersensitive proprioceptor activity. Counterstrain treatment uses precise body positioning to reduce the hypersensitive muscle spindle activity and abnormal muscle contractions of the dysfunctional muscle.
ME	Direct or indirect	Active	*Postisometric relaxation* During the patient's contraction, increased pressure is placed on the Golgi tendon organ proprioceptors within the muscle tendon. This leads to reflex inhibition and subsequent muscle lengthening. *Reciprocal inhibition* Uses the agonist/antagonist relationship of inverse relaxation with contraction *Respiratory assistance* Uses patient's respirations to move soma through a barrier *Joint mobilization* Use of muscular attachments and physician's hands as fulcrums to mobilize joints with limited mobility
HVLA	Direct	Passive	A technique employing a rapid, therapeutic force of brief duration that travels a short distance within the anatomic range of motion of a joint. It engages the restrictive barrier of an articular somatic dysfunction in one or more planes of motion to elicit release of restriction. Sometimes, an audible cavitational pop can be heard which has been described as release of entrapped synovial folds/gas or articular adhesions within a joint. HVLA is also known as thrust technique.
OCMM	Either	Passive	(Previously called osteopathy in the cranial field [OCF]) is a system of diagnosis and treatment by an osteopathic physician that uses the primary respiratory mechanism and balanced membranous and ligamentous tension. It refers to the system of diagnosis and treatment first described by William G. Sutherland, DO.

Sympathetic	Parasympathetic	ICD–10 Codes	
T1–T4(5)	Vagus	M99.00	SD Head
T1–T5		M99.01	SD Cervical
T2–T4(5)		M99.02	SD Thoracic
T5–T6		M99.03	SD Lumbar
T6–T10(5–9)		M99.04	SD Sacrum
T7–T9(5–11)		M99.05	SD Pelvis
T(6)7–9		M99.06	SD Lower Extremities
T9–T10(11)	S2–S4	M99.07	SD Upper Extremities
T10–L1		M99.08	SD Rib Cage
T(10)12–L1		M99.09	SD Abdomen/Other
L1–L2			
T(9)10–11		**CPT Areas Treated**	
T(10)11–L2		98925	1–2 areas
T(10)12–L1		98926	3–4 areas
T2–T5(7)		98927	5–6 areas
T(10)11–L2(3)		98928	7–8 areas
		98929	9–10 areas

Continued

Anterior Chapman's Points

Area	Anterior Points
Middle ear	Superior clavicular border 1/3 from midline
Sinuses	Inferior clavicular border 1/3 from midline
Myocardium	2nd ICS
Esophagus	2nd ICS
Thyroid	2nd ICS
Bronchi	2nd ICS
Upper lung	3rd ICS
Lower lung	4th ICS
Liver	5th and 6th ICS R
Stomach	5th and 6th ICS L
Gallbladder	6th ICS R
Pancreas	7th ICS R
Spleen	7th ICS L
Appendix	Tip of the 12th rib R
Adrenals	1 inch lateral and 2 inches superior to umbilicus
Kidneys	1 inch lateral and 1 inch superior to umbilicus
Bladder	Periumbilical area
Ovaries, urethra	Superior pubic ramus, 2 cm lateral to symphysis
Prostate	Outer femur (along posterior ITB) bilateral
Pylorus	Center of sternum

Prevertebral Ganglia (Collateral Ganglia)

Celiac ganglion	Just below xiphoid process	Esophagus, stomach, duodenum
Superior mesenteric ganglion	Between points for the celiac and inferior mesenteric ganglion	Jejunum to transverse colon
Inferior mesenteric ganglion	Just above the umbilicus	Descending colon to rectum

ªPatient refusal or lack of somatic dysfunction is always a contraindication.

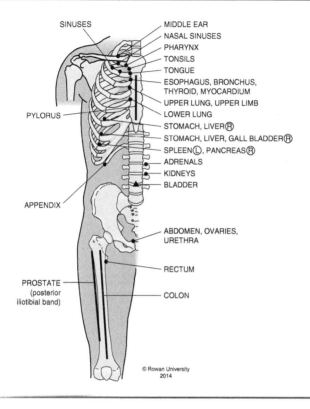

SINUSES

MIDDLE EAR
NASAL SINUSES
PHARYNX
TONSILS
TONGUE
ESOPHAGUS, BRONCHUS,
THYROID, MYOCARDIUM
UPPER LUNG, UPPER LIMB
LOWER LUNG
STOMACH, LIVER(R)
STOMACH, LIVER, GALL BLADDER(R)
SPLEEN(L), PANCREAS(R)
ADRENALS
KIDNEYS
BLADDER

PYLORUS

APPENDIX

ABDOMEN, OVARIES,
URETHRA

RECTUM

PROSTATE
(posterior
iliotibial band)

COLON

© Rowan University
2014

CONTENTS

SECTION I: DIAGNOSES

CONTENTS

SECTION II: STRUCTURAL EVALUATIONS AND TREATMENT TECHNIQUES

DIAGNOSING SOMATIC DYSFUNCTION

FOCUSED STRUCTURAL EXAMS

TECHNIQUES

Head

CONTENTS

Lumbar

Sacrum

Innominate

Upper Extremity

CONTENTS

CONTENTS

SUMMARY CHARTS

ACRONYMS AND ABBREVIATIONS

AA	atlantoaxial
Abd	abdomen
ART	articulatory
ASIS	anterior superior iliac spine
Attn	attention
BLT	balanced ligamentous tension
CN	cranial nerve
CPT	Current Procedural Terminology
CR	cranial sacral technique
CRI	cranial rhythmic impulse
CS	counterstrain
CV4	fourth cerebral ventricle
DIR	direct inhibition
FABERE	Flexion, ABduction, External Rotation, and Extension C
FPR	facilitated positional release
GERD	gastroesophageal reflux disease
GI	gastrointestinal (tract)
HVLA	high velocity/low amplitude
IBD	inflammatory bowel disease
IBS	irritable bowel syndrome
ICS	intercostal space
ILAs	inferior lateral angles
ITB	iliotibial band
LE	lower extremity
m.	muscle
MCP	metacarpophalangeal
MET	muscle energy technique
MFR	myofascial release
mm.	muscles
n.	nerve
nn.	nerves
OA	occipitoatlantoid
OCMM	osteopathic cranial manipulative medicine
OM	occipitomastoid
OMM	osteopathic manipulative medicine
OMT	osteopathic manipulative treatment
PINS	progressive inhibition of neuromuscular structures
PSIS	posterior superior iliac spine
SBS	sphenobasilar synchondrosis
SCM	sternocleidomastoid
SD	somatic dysfunction

Continued

ACRONYMS AND ABBREVIATIONS *Continued*

SI	sacroiliac
ST	soft tissue
SPG	sphenopalatine ganglion
TMJ	used for temporomandibular joint *and* temporomandibular joint dysfunction
TNF-α	tumor necrosis factor-α
TPI	trigger point injection
Tx	treatment
UE	upper extremity
VIS	visceral technique

Section I
Diagnoses

ALLERGY/POSTNASAL DRIP

 BASICS

DESCRIPTION

Inflammation of the nasal passages and upper airway secondary to immune response to allergens

 PHYSIOLOGY AND ASSOCIATED SOMATIC DYSFUNCTIONS

PARASYMPATHETICS

- Increased tone = significantly increased secretions of nasal, lacrimal, and submandibular glands
- Facial (CN VII), glossopharyngeal (CN IX)—cranial dysfunction
- Vagus nerve (CN X)
  - ➤ Somatic dysfunctions of occipitoatlantal joint (OA), atlantoaxial joint (AA), C2
  - ➤ Compression of occipitomastoid sutures as well as occipitoatlantal joint

SYMPATHETICS

- Increased tone = vasoconstriction and slight secretions of nasal, lacrimal, and submandibular glands
- Somatic dysfunctions of T1–T4 (head and neck). Head and neck sympathetics arise from upper thoracic region and return through cervical ganglion.

MOTOR

- Somatic dysfunctions of C3–C5 (phrenic nerve to the diaphragm; irritation because of lung proximity and cough)

 OTHER SOMATIC DYSFUNCTIONS

- Eustachian tube dysfunction
- Cranial dysfunction
- Lymphatic congestion of lymph nodes: preauricular and postauricular, submaxillary and submental, supraclavicular
- Anterior fascial restriction of the cervical region down into sternum with resulting tenderpoints
- Rib dysfunction

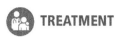

TREATMENT

2-MINUTE TREATMENT

- Head—supraorbital (CN V1), infraorbital (CN V2), mental (CN V3): nerve stimulation **M99.00**
- Cervical (OA, AA, C2): MFR, ST, FPR, or MET **M99.01**
- Head—nasion gapping **M99.00**

5-MINUTE TREATMENT

- Head—sphenopalatine ganglion stimulation **M99.00**
- Head—Muncie technique **M99.00**
- Head—periauricular drainage technique **M99.00**
- Head—Galbreath technique (mandibular drainage) **M99.00**

EXTENDED TREATMENT

- Thoracic—left thoracic duct: lymphatic **M99.02**
- Head—vagus: OA release **M99.00**
- Cervical—anterior cervical: MFR **M99.01**
- Thoracic—MET, MFR, and/or HVLA **M99.02**
- Rib dysfunction—MET **M99.08**
- Abdomen—diaphragm
  - ➤ Doming technique **M99.09**
  - ➤ Thoracolumbar junction—MET, MFR, HVLA **M99.02**, **M99.03**
- Abdomen/other/viscerosomatic—Chapman's reflex for ear and/or sinuses **M99.09**

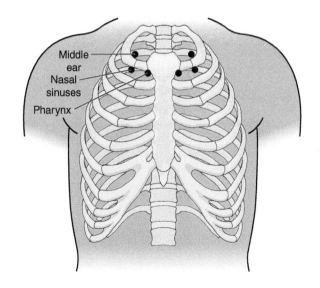

ANKLE SPRAIN

 BASICS

DESCRIPTION

A nonphysiological stretching or twisting of the ankle joint resulting in tears of its ligaments or other soft tissue

 PHYSIOLOGY AND ASSOCIATED SOMATIC DYSFUNCTIONS

PARASYMPATHETICS

Not applicable

SYMPATHETICS

- Increased tone = dilated arterioles of the muscles (cholinergic and adrenergic β2), constricted arterioles of the muscles (adrenergic α)
- Somatic dysfunctions of T10–L2

MOTOR

- L4–S2 common fibular nerve
  - ➤ Impinged by posterior fibular head somatic dysfunction
- Tenderness and/or edema of any of the following:
  - ➤ Lateral ankle (inversion sprain) L4–S2 superficial fibular nerve
    - → Fibularis/peroneus longus muscle and tendon
    - → Fibularis/peroneus brevis muscle and tendon
  - ➤ Medial ankle (eversion sprain) L4–S3 tibial nerve
    - → Flexor hallucis longus muscle and tendon
    - → Flexor digitorum longus muscle and tendon
    - → Tibialis posterior muscle and tendon
  - ➤ Posterior ankle L4–S3 tibial nerve
    - → Soleus muscle and tendon
    - → Gastrocnemius muscle and tendon

 OTHER SOMATIC DYSFUNCTIONS

- Hind foot restrictions—calcaneus and talus
- Midfoot restrictions—navicular, cuneiform, and cuboid
- Forefoot restrictions—metatarsals
- Posterior and inferior fibular head (with inversion sprain)
- Anterior tibia on talus

TREATMENT

 2-MINUTE TREATMENT

- Lower extremity—direct MFR (soft tissue) stretching of associated muscles **M99.06**

 5-MINUTE TREATMENT

- Lower extremity—strain-counterstrain for tenderpoints of associated muscle and tendons CS **M99.06**
- Lower extremity—lymphatic drainage of ankle edema: gentle effleurage **M99.06**
- Lower extremity—posterior fibular head: CS, MET, and/or HVLA **M99.06**

 EXTENDED TREATMENT

- Lower extremity—anterior tibia on talus: articulatory technique **M99.06**
- Lower extremity—somatic dysfunctions of foot; ART, BLT, and/or CS **M99.06**

ANXIETY

 BASICS

DESCRIPTION

An acute or chronic fearful emotion often with associated physical symptoms

 PHYSIOLOGY AND ASSOCIATED SOMATIC DYSFUNCTIONS

PARASYMPATHETICS

- Increased tone = decreased heart rate, increased acid secretion, nausea, vomiting, bowel motility/diarrhea, increased bladder contraction
  - ➤ Vagus nerve (CN X) exits the jugular foramen (composed of occiput and temporal bones).
    - ➜ Somatic dysfunctions of occipitoatlantal joint (OA), atlantoaxial joint (AA), C2
    - ➜ Compression of occipitomastoid sutures

SYMPATHETICS

- Increased tone = tachycardia, increased sensitivity to acid, decreased bowel motility/constipation, decreased bladder contraction
  - ➤ Somatic dysfunctions of T1–T4 (cardiac) and/or T5–L2 (gastrointestinal)
  - ➤ Fascial restriction of prevertebral ganglion: celiac, superior mesenteric, and inferior mesenteric ganglion

MOTOR

- Somatic dysfunctions of C2–C7 (levator scapulae muscle, scalene muscle, upper trapezius muscle, posterior cervical musculature)

 OTHER SOMATIC DYSFUNCTIONS

- TMJ dysfunction
  - ➤ Medial and lateral pterygoid muscle hypertonicity
- Upper cross syndrome
  - ➤ Trigger points and hypertonicity of upper trapezius muscle, levator scapulae muscle, sternocleidomastoid muscle, and pectoralis muscles
- Inhalation dysfunctions of ribs 1 and 2

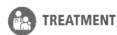

TREATMENT

2-MINUTE TREATMENT

- Upper extremity—trapezius muscle release DIR **M99.07**

5-MINUTE TREATMENT

- Head
  - ➤ OA release **M99.00**
  - ➤ Cranial strains OCMM **M99.00**
  - ➤ V spread for OM somatic dysfunction **M99.00**
  - ➤ TMJ—pterygoid release DIR **M99.00**
- Cervical—FPR **M99.01**

EXTENDED TREATMENT

- Head—abnormal cranial strain pattern: treat strain **M99.00**
  - ➤ Vault hold
  - ➤ CV4 hold
- Cervical—C2–C7: MET, MFR, FPR, and/or HVLA **M99.01**
- Upper extremity—muscles of upper cross syndrome: MFR, MET, and/or CS **M99.07**
- Thoracic—MET, MFR, and/or HVLA **M99.02**
- Rib—MET, FPR to inhalation dysfunction of first and second rib **M99.08**
- Lumbar—MET, MFR, and/or HVLA **M99.03**
- Abdomen/other/viscerosomatic
  - ➤ Ganglion restriction: MFR **M99.09**
  - ➤ Mesenteric release: VIS **M99.09**
  - ➤ Chapman's reflex at ITB and other GI and cardiac points as needed **M99.09**

Continued

ANXIETY

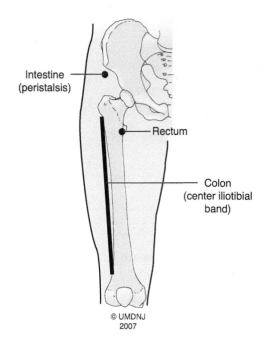

Intestine
(peristalsis)

Rectum

Colon
(center iliotibial
band)

© UMDNJ
2007

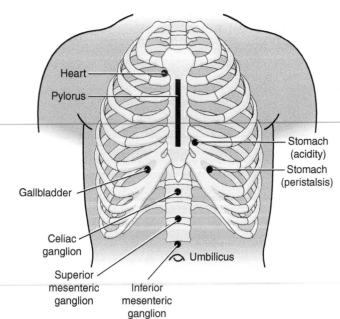

Heart

Pylorus

Stomach
(acidity)

Stomach
(peristalsis)

Gallbladder

Celiac
ganglion

Umbilicus

Superior
mesenteric
ganglion

Inferior
mesenteric
ganglion

ARTHRITIS (INFLAMMATORY)

 BASICS

DESCRIPTION

There are many rheumatologic conditions that can lead to arthritis; the correct diagnosis will direct the appropriate medical management of the patient with joint pain. These recommendations may be helpful to follow during the workup and after the disease has been identified.

 PHYSIOLOGY AND ASSOCIATED SOMATIC DYSFUNCTIONS

PARASYMPATHETICS

- Undetermined
  - ➤ Afferent vagus nerve fibers can be stimulated by endotoxin or cytokines. These can activate the HPA axis and sympathetic nervous system, which can release anti-inflammatory glucocorticoids. The vagus nerve may also inhibit TNF-α production by splenic macrophages.

SYMPATHETICS

- Regulatory function of the sympathetic nervous system (SNS) includes monitoring and influencing immune homeostasis.
- Increased tone
  - ➤ Stimulates catecholamine production in the different lymphoid organs via the efferent fibers, inhibits the development of a Th1 immune response, and shifts the Th1/Th2 balance toward a Th2 immune response, which is "humoral immunity" upregulation of antibody production to fight extracellular organisms
  - ➤ Dilated arterioles of the muscles (cholinergic and adrenergic β2), constricted arterioles of the muscles (adrenergic α)
- Somatic dysfunctions of T5–T7—upper extremity
- Somatic dysfunctions of T10–L2—lower extremity

MOTOR

- Somatic dysfunctions of C4–T1—upper extremity
- Somatic dysfunctions of L1–S3—lower extremity

 OTHER SOMATIC DYSFUNCTIONS

- Any joint may be affected depending on the nature of the rheumatologic condition. Synovitis, bursitis, or generalized edema may accompany the arthritis and may respond to lymphatic drainage techniques.
- Sacroiliitis is common with some rheumatic diseases. The sacrum, innominates, and lumbar spine should be assessed for somatic dysfunction in these individuals. Compensatory findings or overuse syndromes of areas not affected by arthritis should also be evaluated.

TREATMENT

Caution: Inflammatory arthritis may lead to joint instability as a result of ligamentous laxity; therefore, avoidance of HVLA techniques to the upper cervical spine is recommended.

 2-MINUTE TREATMENT

● Thoracic—MET, MFR, and/or HVLA **M99.02**

 5-MINUTE TREATMENT

● Head
  ➤ OA release **M99.00**
  ➤ V spread technique for OM suture somatic dysfunction **M99.00**

 EXTENDED TREATMENT

● Lymphatic effleurage to affected joints **M99.01–M99.08**
● BLT to affected joints **M99.01–M99.08**
● MFR to joints of subjective complaint or objective findings **M99.01–M99.08**
● Strain-counterstrain for tenderpoints of associated joints, muscle, and tendons CS **M99.01–M99.08**

BILLING BY REGION TREATED

● Head/cranial somatic dysfunction **M99.00**
● Cervical somatic dysfunction **M99.01**
● Thoracic somatic dysfunction **M99.02**
● Lumbar somatic dysfunction **M99.03**
● Sacral somatic dysfunction **M99.04**
● Innominate somatic dysfunction **M99.05**
● Lower extremity somatic dysfunction **M99.06**
● Upper extremity somatic dysfunction **M99.07**
● Rib somatic dysfunction **M99.08**
● Abdominal/viscerosomatic dysfunction **M99.09**

ARTHRITIS (OSTEOARTHRITIS)

 BASICS

DESCRIPTION

A noninflammatory degenerative joint disease of any joint in the body, commonly of hands, knees, hips, and spine. It is identified by joint space narrowing, articular derangement as a result of cartilaginous breakdown, and calcium deposition based on Wolff law associated with pain, stiffness, tenderness, joint effusion, crepitus, and reduced range of motion.

 PHYSIOLOGY AND ASSOCIATED SOMATIC DYSFUNCTIONS

PARASYMPATHETICS

Not applicable

SYMPATHETICS

- Dilated arterioles of the muscles (cholinergic and adrenergic β2), constricted arterioles of the muscles (adrenergic α)
- Somatic dysfunctions of T5–T7—upper extremity
- Somatic dysfunctions of T10–L2—lower extremity

MOTOR

- Somatic dysfunctions of C4–T1—upper extremity
- Somatic dysfunctions of L1–S3—lower extremity

 OTHER SOMATIC DYSFUNCTIONS

- Any joint may be affected. History of trauma or repetitive use may localize.
- Cervical, thoracic, lumbar, and sacral arthritis may lead to foraminal or central canal stenosis with the expected associated findings.
- Hands (especially thumbs), knees, and hips are especially prone to osteoarthritis because of gravitational forces and overuse.
- Examine patient for compensatory findings or overuse syndromes of areas not affected by arthritis.

TREATMENT

Note: Treatment should be focused on the restoration and maintenance of function of affected joints. This should include preventive health of the surrounding joints through exercise prescription, postural education, ergonomic evaluation, and recommendations.

 2-MINUTE TREATMENT

- MFR to areas of subjective complaint or objective findings

 5-MINUTE TREATMENT

- Strain-counterstrain to tenderpoints encountered **M99.01–M99.08**

 EXTENDED TREATMENT

- Thoracic—MET, MFR, and/or HVLA **M99.02**
- MFR, MET, or HVLA to areas above and below affected joints
- BLT to affected joints **M99.01–M99.08**
- Ergonomic evaluation and recommendations
- Postural education
- Exercise prescription

BILLING BY REGION TREATED

- Cervical somatic dysfunction **M99.01**
- Thoracic somatic dysfunction **M99.02**
- Lumbar somatic dysfunction **M99.03**
- Sacral somatic dysfunction **M99.04**
- Innominate somatic dysfunction **M99.05**
- Lower extremity somatic dysfunction **M99.06**
- Upper extremity somatic dysfunction **M99.07**

ASTHMA

BASICS

DESCRIPTION

An inflammatory disorder of the tracheobronchial tree characterized by mild to severe obstruction to airflow. The clinical hallmark is wheezing, but cough may be the predominant symptom.

PHYSIOLOGY AND ASSOCIATED SOMATIC DYSFUNCTIONS

PARASYMPATHETICS

- Increased tone = increased volume of secretions and relative bronchiole constriction
- Vagus nerve
  - ➤ Somatic dysfunctions of occipitoatlantal joint (OA), atlantoaxial joint (AA), C2, cranial and cervical dysfunction
  - ➤ Clavicle dysfunction
  - ➤ Compression of occipitomastoid sutures at jugular foramen as well as occipitoatlantoid joint

SYMPATHETICS

- Increased tone = decreased secretions and bronchiole dilation
- Somatic dysfunctions of T2–T7

MOTOR

- Somatic dysfunctions of C3–C5 (phrenic nerve to the diaphragm; dysfunction as a result of decreased excursion and overuse)
- Anterior cervical soft tissue (anterior scalene muscle) dysfunction
- Rib 1 dysfunction
- Clavicle dysfunction

OTHER SOMATIC DYSFUNCTIONS

- Cranial vault dysfunction
- Anterior and middle scalene muscles—ribs 1
- Posterior scalene muscles—ribs 2
- Sternocleidomastoid muscle—clavicle
- Inhalation or exhalation dysfunction of ribs
- Diaphragm dysfunction or attachments to xiphoid process, inferior ribs, and lumbar spine (L1–L3)

TREATMENT

 2-MINUTE TREATMENT

- Cervical—ST **M99.01**
- Thoracic—ST, seated MET **M99.02**

 5-MINUTE TREATMENT

- Upper extremity—pectoralis minor muscle: CS, MFR, and/or pectoralis muscle traction (for lymphatic treatment) **M99.07**
- Thoracic—HVLA **M99.02**
- Rib dysfunction—MET **M99.08**
- Rib raising **M99.08**

 EXTENDED TREATMENT

- Head—CV4 **M99.00**
- Head—OA release **M99.00**
- Cervical—C2, C3–C5: soft tissue, MET, and/or HVLA **M99.01**
- Cervical—scalene muscles: CS and/or MET **M99.01**
- Abdominal diaphragm
  - ➤ Diaphragm doming technique **M99.09**
  - ➤ Lumbar—soft tissue, MET, and/or HVLA **M99.03**

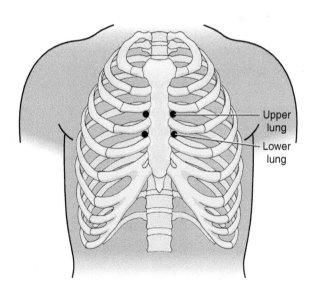

Upper lung
Lower lung

ATELECTASIS

 BASICS

DESCRIPTION

A condition in which the lung, in whole or in part, is collapsed or without air and the alveoli are collapsed. It implies some blockage of a bronchiole or bronchus, which can be within the airway (foreign body, mucus plug), from the wall (tumor, usually squamous cell carcinoma), or compressing from the outside (tumor, lymph node).

 PHYSIOLOGY AND ASSOCIATED SOMATIC DYSFUNCTIONS

PARASYMPATHETICS

- Increased tone = increased secretions and relative bronchiole constriction
- Vagus nerve
  - ➤ Somatic dysfunctions of occipitoatlantal joint (OA), atlantoaxial joint (AA), C2, cranial and cervical dysfunction
  - ➤ Compression of occipitomastoid sutures as well as occipitoatlantoid joint

SYMPATHETICS

- Increased tone = decreased secretions and bronchiole dilation
- Somatic dysfunctions of T2–T7

MOTOR

- Somatic dysfunctions of C3–C5 (phrenic nerve to the diaphragm; dysfunction as a result of decreased excursion and overuse), cervical dysfunction

 OTHER SOMATIC DYSFUNCTIONS

- Ribs dysfunctions
- Thoracoabdominal diaphragm somatic dysfunction

A

 TREATMENT

 2-MINUTE TREATMENT

- Thoracic lymphatic pump (thoracic SD) **M99.02**

 5-MINUTE TREATMENT

- Rib raising **M99.08**
- Thoracic—MFR and/or ST **M99.02**
- Abdomen—diaphragm
  - ➤ Doming technique **M99.09**
  - ➤ Thoracolumbar junction: MET, MFR, ST, and HVLA **M99.02**, **M99.03**
  - ➤ Costochondral margin and xiphoid process: CS, MFR **M99.08**

 EXTENDED TREATMENT

- Rib dysfunction—MET **M99.08**
- Cervical—C2, C3–C5: MFR, ST, MET, and/or FPR **M99.01**
- Head—vagus: OA release and/or V spread **M99.00**
- Abdomen and other viscerosomatic reflexes—Chapman's reflex for lung **M99.09**

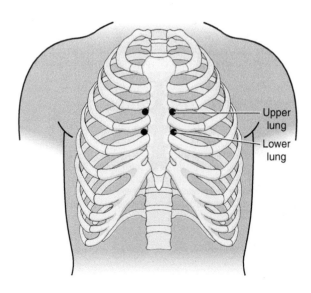

Upper lung

Lower lung

BELL'S PALSY

 ## BASICS

DESCRIPTION

A form of unilateral facial paralysis resulting from inflammation, trauma, or entrapment one of the facial nerves (CN VII)

 ## PHYSIOLOGY AND ASSOCIATED SOMATIC DYSFUNCTIONS

PARASYMPATHETICS

- Because the parasympathetic fibers to the lacrimal gland and the submandibular gland separate from CN VII prior to exiting the stylomastoid foramen, these functions should be unaffected. However, irritation of the nerve may reflexively cause dysfunction of these glands, stimulating secretion from the submandibular, sublingual, and lacrimal glands as well as the mucous membranes of the nasopharynx and hard and soft palates.
- CN VII
  - ➤ Cranial dysfunctions, especially of the temporal bones
  - ➤ Compression of occipitomastoid sutures

SYMPATHETICS

- Inhibit secretion from the submandibular, sublingual, and lacrimal glands as well as the mucous membranes of the nasopharynx and hard and soft palates
- Somatic dysfunctions T1–T4

MOTOR

- CN VII—muscles of facial expression, including frontalis and orbicularis oculi, muscles of the nasolabial folds, labial muscles, buccal muscles, posterior belly of the digastric muscles, and the platysma muscle, will all be paralyzed on the affected side.

 ## OTHER SOMATIC DYSFUNCTIONS

- Somatic dysfunction of temporal bones
- Somatic dysfunction of occipital bone
- Somatic dysfunction of posterior digastric muscle
- TMJ—medial pterygoid muscles, glossal muscles, hyoid muscles, and fascial restrictions
- Sternocleidomastoid muscle hypertonicity (due to attachment to temporal bone)
- Any cervical dysfunction related to muscular attachments
- Lymphatic congestion of lymph nodes: preauricular and postauricular, submaxillary and submental, supraclavicular

TREATMENT

 2-MINUTE TREATMENT

- Head—Galbreath technique (mandibular drainage) **M99.00**

 5-MINUTE TREATMENT

- Head—cranial dysfunction (especially temporal dysfunction): vault hold/cranial treatment **M99.00**

 EXTENDED TREATMENT

- Head—OA release **M99.00**
- Head—compressed occipitomastoid suture: V spread **M99.00**
- Head—decreased CRI: CV4 hold **M99.00**
- Cervical—FPR, MET, MFR, and/or ST **M99.01**
- Thoracic—T1–T4: MET, MFR, and/or HVLA **M99.02**
- Head—TMJ: direct inhibition or CS to tenderpoints **M99.00**
- Thoracic inlet—MFR **M99.02**
- Abdomen—respiratory diaphragm: doming **M99.09**

CARPAL TUNNEL SYNDROME

 BASICS

Often a painful peripheral neuropathic condition of the hand and wrist accompanied by paresthesias and weakness in the distribution of the median nerve distal to the wrist; caused by compression of the median nerve as it passes through the carpal tunnel

 PHYSIOLOGY AND ASSOCIATED SOMATIC DYSFUNCTIONS

PARASYMPATHETICS

Not applicable

SYMPATHETICS

- Increased tone = dilated arterioles of the muscles (cholinergic and adrenergic β2), constricted arterioles of the muscles (adrenergic α)
- Somatic dysfunctions of T5–T7

MOTOR

- Median nerve (C5–T1)—distal to the wrist innervates the opponens pollicis muscle, superficial head of flexor pollicis brevis muscle, and first two lumbricals. Dermatomal pattern—palmar surface; distal first digit; second, third, and lateral half of fourth digit
  - ➤ Displaced carpal bones
  - ➤ Edema of the distal upper extremity

 OTHER SOMATIC DYSFUNCTIONS

- Somatic dysfunction of flexor retinaculum (transverse carpal ligament)
- Interosseous membrane tenderpoints and fascial restrictions
- Carpal bones: lunate and capitate anterior somatic dysfunction
- Hypertonicity of forearm flexor muscles

Note: Rule out cervical radiculopathy and thoracic outlet syndrome.

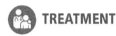 **TREATMENT**

 2-MINUTE TREATMENT

- Upper extremity—flexor retinaculum: MFR **M99.07**

 5-MINUTE TREATMENT

- Upper extremity—carpal bone: BLT, MET, and HVLA **M99.07**
- Thoracic—HVLA **M99.02**

 EXTENDED TREATMENT

- Cervical—C5–T1: FPR, MFR, and/or HVLA **M99.01**
- Thoracic—FPR, MFR, and/or MET **M99.02**
- Upper extremity—interosseous membrane BLT: forearm flexor muscles CS, MFR **M99.07**

C

CERVICAL SPONDYLOSIS

BASICS

DESCRIPTION

A condition of the intervertebral disks and the surrounding bony vertebrae in the cervical spine that most likely is caused by degenerative changes

PHYSIOLOGY AND ASSOCIATED SOMATIC DYSFUNCTIONS

PARASYMPATHETICS

Not applicable

SYMPATHETICS

- Increased tone = dilated arterioles of the muscles (cholinergic and adrenergic β2), constricted arterioles of the muscles (adrenergic α)
- Somatic dysfunctions T1–T5 (Sympathetic tone to the head and neck arises from thoracic spine and returns cephalad through the cervical ganglion.)

MOTOR

- Somatic dysfunctions C1–C8—nerve roots, spinal accessory nerve (CN XI): levator scapula muscle, longus capitis, longus colli muscle, scalene muscles, splenius muscle, sternocleidomastoid muscle, rectus capitis muscle

OTHER SOMATIC DYSFUNCTIONS

- OA
- AA, C2–C7
- Scalene muscle hypertonicity, tenderpoints, and restricted motion
- Inhalation dysfunction of ribs 1 and 2
- Clavicle somatic dysfunction
- Pectoralis minor muscle hypertonicity, tenderpoints, and restricted motion
- Levator scapulae muscle hypertonicity, tenderpoints, and restricted motion
- Rhomboid muscle hypertonicity, tenderpoints, and restricted motion
- Teres major muscle, teres minor muscle, and latissimus dorsi muscle tenderpoints and hypertonicity (posterior axillary region)

TREATMENT

 2-MINUTE TREATMENT

- Head—OA release **M99.00**
- Cervical—FPR, MFR, and/or ST **M99.01**

 5-MINUTE TREATMENT

- Ribs 1 and 2—FPR and/or MET **M99.08**
- Cervical—MET **M99.01**

 EXTENDED TREATMENT

- Thoracic—MET, FPR, MFR, and/or ST **M99.02**
- Upper extremity—pectoralis minor muscle: CS, MET **M99.07**
- Cervical—scalene muscles: MET, CS **M99.01**
- Upper extremity—levator scapulae muscle: CS, MET **M99.07**
- Upper extremity—rhomboid muscle: CS, MET **M99.07**
- Upper extremity—clavicle: MFR, MET **M99.07**
- Upper extremity—posterior axillary region tenderpoints and hypertonicity: CS **M99.07**

C

CHOLECYSTITIS

 BASICS

DESCRIPTION

Inflammation of the gallbladder

 PHYSIOLOGY AND ASSOCIATED SOMATIC DYSFUNCTIONS

PARASYMPATHETICS

- Increased tone = contraction of gallbladder and bile ducts
- Vagus nerve (CN X) exits the jugular foramen (composed of occiput and temporal bones).
  - ➤ Somatic dysfunctions of occipitoatlantal joint (OA), atlantoaxial joint (AA), C2
  - ➤ Compression of occipitomastoid sutures

SYMPATHETICS

- Increased tone = relaxation of gallbladder and bile ducts
- Somatic dysfunctions of T5–T9
- Celiac ganglion fascial restriction

MOTOR

- Somatic dysfunctions of C3–C5 (phrenic nerve to the diaphragm; dysfunction as a result of diaphragm irritation)

 OTHER SOMATIC DYSFUNCTIONS

- Diaphragm—restriction of gross motion and at all attachments
- Mid and lower rib dysfunction as a result of splinting
- Celiac ganglion fascial restriction
- Thoracic outlet—clavicle, first rib, scalene muscles, T1 (left thoracic duct fascial restriction)
- Cisterna chyli—fascial restriction
- Mesenteric fascial restriction

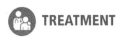 **TREATMENT**

 2-MINUTE TREATMENT

● Thoracic—seated MET **M99.02**

 5-MINUTE TREATMENT

● Rib raising **M99.08**
● Abdomen—mesenteric release: MFR **M99.09**

 EXTENDED TREATMENT

● Head—vagus nerve: OA release, MFR; pterygoid release, DIR **M99.00**
● Cervical—C2; C3–C5: MFR, FPR, and/or HVLA **M99.01**
● Thoracic—T5–T9: BLT, MFR, and/or HVLA **M99.02**
● Abdomen—cisterna chyli and thoracic duct (lymphatic) **M99.09**
● Abdomen—diaphragm: doming **M99.09**
● Abdomen—liver pump **M99.09**
● Abdomen—celiac ganglion release VIS **M99.09**
● Abdomen/other/viscerosomatic—Chapman's reflex for gallbladder and liver **M99.09**
● Rib dysfunction—MET **M99.08**
● Ribs—diaphragm attachments (costal margins, xyphoid **M99.08**, T12/L1 **M99.03**): BLT, MFR **M99.08**

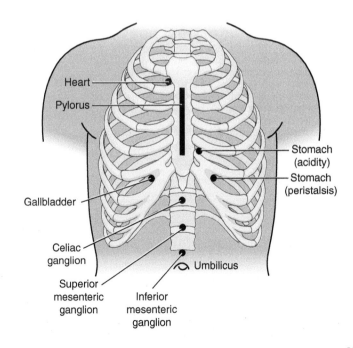

CHRONIC OBSTRUCTIVE PULMONARY DISEASE

 BASICS

DESCRIPTION

Used to describe emphysema (the destruction of interalveolar septa) and chronic bronchitis (increased mucus production and chronic cough); characterized by airflow reduction that is not fully reversible with bronchodilators

 PHYSIOLOGY AND ASSOCIATED SOMATIC DYSFUNCTIONS

PARASYMPATHETICS

- Increased tone = thinning of secretions and relative bronchiole constriction
- Vagus nerve
  - Somatic dysfunctions of occipitoatlantal joint (OA), atlantoaxial joint (AA), C2, head and cervical dysfunction

SYMPATHETICS

- Increased tone = thickened secretions and bronchiole dilation
  - Somatic dysfunctions of T2–T7

MOTOR

- Somatic dysfunctions of C3–C5 (phrenic nerve to the diaphragm as a result of decreased excursion and overuse), cervical dysfunction

 OTHER SOMATIC DYSFUNCTIONS

- Scalene muscle hypertonicity and tenderpoints
- Sternocleidomastoid muscle hypertonicity and tenderpoints
- Pectoralis minor muscle hypertonicity and tenderpoints
- Serratus anterior muscle hypertonicity and tenderpoints
- Inhalation-type rib dysfunctions
- Thoracic inlet diaphragm dysfunctions
- Flattened diaphragm with decreased excursion

TREATMENT

 2-MINUTE TREATMENT

- Head—OA release **M99.00**
- Cervical—ST or MFR **M99.01**
- Thoracic—ST or MFR **M99.02**

 5-MINUTE TREATMENT

- Thoracic—MET or HVLA **M99.02**
- Rib—MET **M99.08**
- Abdomen—diaphragm: doming technique **M99.09**

 EXTENDED TREATMENT

- Thoracolumbar—ST, MFR, and MET **M99.02**, **M99.03**
- Cervical—MET, HVLA, or FPR **M99.01**
- Cervical—scalene muscle: CS or MET **M99.01**
- Cervical—sternocleidomastoid muscle: CS, MFR, or MET **M99.01**
- Upper extremity—pectoralis minor muscle: CS or MET **M99.07**
- Thoracic—serratus anterior muscle: CS or MET **M99.02**
- Thoracic inlet release—MFR **M99.02**
- Abdomen/other/viscerosomatic—Chapman's reflex for lung **M99.09**

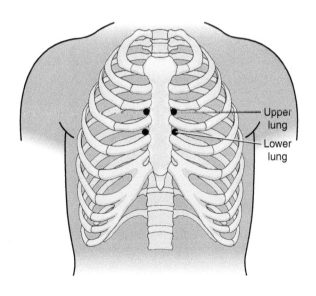

Upper lung
Lower lung

COLIC

 ## BASICS

DESCRIPTION

Characterized by irritable children who are not easily consolable and are poor sleepers and poor eaters; excessively gassy and shows other signs of gastric discomfort; diagnosis of exclusion and medical conditions needs to be ruled out.

 ## PHYSIOLOGY AND ASSOCIATED SOMATIC DYSFUNCTIONS

PARASYMPATHETICS

- Increased tone = thinning of secretions, relative bronchiole constriction, and increased peristalsis
- Facial nerve (CN VII)
- Vagus nerve (CN X) exits the jugular foramen (composed of occiput and temporal bones).
  - ➤ Somatic dysfunctions of occipitoatlantal joint (OA), atlantoaxial joint (AA), C2
  - ➤ Compression of occipitomastoid sutures

SYMPATHETICS

- Increased tone = thickened secretions, bronchiole dilation, decreased peristalsis
- Somatic dysfunctions of T1–L2
- Celiac, superior, and inferior mesenteric ganglia restrictions

 ## OTHER SOMATIC DYSFUNCTIONS

- Thoracolumbar dysfunctions
- Respiratory diaphragm dysfunction and at all attachments
- Cranial dysfunctions
- Occipital condylar compression

TREATMENT

 2-MINUTE TREATMENT

- Thoracic and lumbar spine—MFR **M99.02**, **M99.03**
- Head—OA decompression **M99.00**

 5-MINUTE TREATMENT

- Abdomen—diaphragm release: BLT **M99.09**
- Sacrum—sacral release **M99.04**

 EXTENDED TREATMENT

- Cervical—MFR **M99.01**
- Abdomen—ganglion restriction: MFR **M99.09**
- Head—cranial dysfunctions
  - ➤ CV4 **M99.00**
  - ➤ Vault hold **M99.00**
- Condylar decompression **M99.00**

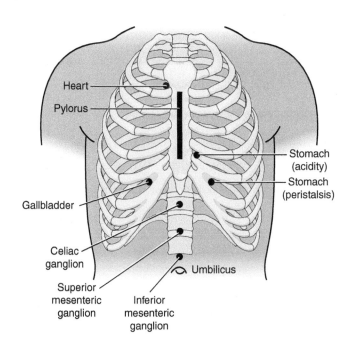

COMMON COLD

 BASICS

DESCRIPTION

Inflammation of the nasal passages and upper airway secondary to respiratory viruses

 PHYSIOLOGY AND ASSOCIATED SOMATIC DYSFUNCTIONS

PARASYMPATHETICS

- Increased tone = significantly increased secretions of nasal, lacrimal, and submandibular glands
- Facial (CN VII), glossopharyngeal (CN IX)—cranial dysfunction
- Vagus nerve (CN X)
  - ➤ Somatic dysfunctions of occipitoatlantal joint (OA), atlantoaxial joint (AA), C2, cranial and cervical dysfunction
  - ➤ Compression of occipitomastoid sutures as well as occipitoatlantoid joint

SYMPATHETICS

- Increased tone = vasoconstriction and slight secretions of nasal, lacrimal, and submandibular glands
- Somatic dysfunctions of T1–T4—head, neck, and respiratory; thoracic dysfunction (Head and neck sympathetics arise from upper thoracic region and return through cervical ganglion.)

MOTOR

- Somatic dysfunctions of C3–C5 (phrenic nerve to the diaphragm; irritation because of lung proximity), cervical dysfunction
- Oculomotor (CN III, CN VII, CN IX, CN X)—cranial dysfunction

 OTHER SOMATIC DYSFUNCTIONS

- Eustachian tube dysfunction
- Cranial dysfunction
- Lymphatic congestion of lymph nodes: preauricular and postauricular, submaxillary and submental, supraclavicular
- Anterior fascial restriction of the cervical region down into sternum with resulting tenderpoints
- Rib dysfunction

TREATMENT

 2-MINUTE TREATMENT

- Head—periauricular drainage technique **M99.00**
- Head—supraorbital (CN V1), infraorbital (CN V2), mental (CN V3): nerve stimulation **M99.00**
- Head—Galbreath technique (mandibular drainage) **M99.00**

 5-MINUTE TREATMENT

- Head—sphenopalatine ganglion stimulation **M99.00**
- Head—cervical (OA, AA, C2): MFR, ST, FPR, or MET **M99.01**
- Head—Muncie technique **M99.00**
- Head—nasion gapping **M99.00**

 EXTENDED TREATMENT

- Thoracic—left thoracic duct: lymphatic **M99.02**
- Head—vagus: OA release **M99.00**
- Cervical—anterior cervical: MFR **M99.01**
- Abdomen/other—sternum: CS, MFR **M99.08**
- Thoracic—MET, MFR, and/or HVLA **M99.02**
- Rib dysfunction—MET **M99.08**
- Rib raising **M99.08**
- Abdomen—diaphragm
  - ➤ Doming technique **M99.09**
  - ➤ Thoracolumbar junction—MET, MFR, HVLA **M99.02**, **M99.03**
- Abdomen/other/viscerosomatic—Chapman's reflex for ear and/or sinuses **M99.09**

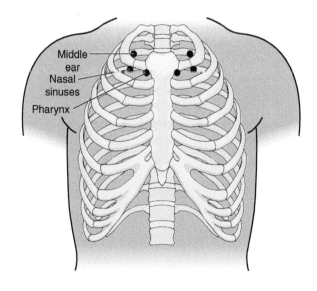

Middle ear
Nasal sinuses
Pharynx

COMPLEX REGIONAL PAIN SYNDROME (REFLEX SYMPATHETIC DYSTROPHY)

 BASICS

DESCRIPTION

A complex of signs and symptoms related to hypersympatheticatonia of one or more extremities characterized by pain, erythema, and edema; commonly following trauma to the affected limb classically not only after a crush injury but also after surgery or other injury

 PHYSIOLOGY AND ASSOCIATED SOMATIC DYSFUNCTIONS

PARASYMPATHETICS

Not applicable; unopposed sympathetic tone to extremities key to this disease process

SYMPATHETICS

- Increased tone = dilated arterioles of the muscles (cholinergic and adrenergic β2), constricted arterioles of the muscles (adrenergic α)
- Somatic dysfunctions of T5–T7—upper extremity: thoracic dysfunction
- Somatic dysfunctions of T10–L2—lower extremity: thoracic and lumbar dysfunction

MOTOR

- Somatic dysfunctions of C4–T1—nerve roots, upper extremity: cervical and thoracic dysfunction
- Somatic dysfunctions of L1–S3—lower extremity: lumbar and sacral dysfunction

 OTHER SOMATIC DYSFUNCTIONS

- Upper and lower extremity lymphedema and fascial strains
- Compensatory findings for antalgic gait or overuse syndromes of areas not directly affected by complex regional pain syndrome

TREATMENT

 2-MINUTE TREATMENT

- Thoracic—ST or MET **M99.02**
- Lumbar—ST or MET **M99.03**

 5-MINUTE TREATMENT

- Cervical—ST, MET, or HVLA **M99.01**
- Thoracic—FPR, MFR, or HVLA **M99.02**
- Lumbar—FPR, MFR, or HVLA **M99.03**
- Sacrum—MET **M99.04**

 EXTENDED TREATMENT

- Upper extremity—MFR, lymphatic **M99.07**
- Lower extremity—MFR, lymphatic **M99.06**
- Rib raising **M99.08**

C

CONGESTIVE HEART FAILURE

 BASICS

DESCRIPTION

A dysfunction of the cardiac pump that results in insufficient blood flow to meet the metabolic requirements of the body

 PHYSIOLOGY AND ASSOCIATED SOMATIC DYSFUNCTIONS

PARASYMPATHETICS

- Increased tone = bradycardia
- Vagus nerve (CN X) exits the jugular foramen (composed of occiput and temporal bones).
  - ➤ Somatic dysfunctions of occipitoatlantal joint (OA), atlantoaxial joint (AA), C2
  - ➤ Compression of occipitomastoid sutures

SYMPATHETICS

- Increased tone = tachycardia
- Somatic dysfunctions of T1–T5

MOTOR

- Somatic dysfunctions of C3–C5 (phrenic nerve to the diaphragm; irritation because of lung proximity)

 OTHER SOMATIC DYSFUNCTIONS

- Dependent extremity edema
- Somatic dysfunction of pelvic floor (diaphragm)
- Somatic dysfunction of popliteal fossa (diaphragm)
- Rib dysfunction
- Flattened diaphragm
- Scalene muscle hypertonicity and tenderpoints
- Pectoralis minor muscle hypertonicity and tenderpoints

TREATMENT

2-MINUTE TREATMENT

- Rib raising **M99.08**

5-MINUTE TREATMENT

- Lower extremity—pedal pump **M99.06**

EXTENDED TREATMENT

- Head—vagus nerve: OA release or V spread **M99.00**
- Head—decreased CRI: CV4 hold **M99.00**
- Cervical—C2, C3–C5: MFR, MET, and/or FPR **M99.01**
- Cervical—scalene muscles: CS or MET **M99.01**
- Thoracic—MFR **M99.02**
- Thoracic—thoracic inlet release BLT **M99.02**
- Rib dysfunction—MET **M99.08**
- Upper extremity—effleurage **M99.07**
- Upper extremity—pectoralis minor muscle: CS or MFR **M99.07**
- Pelvic—pelvic floor muscles release: DIR **M99.05**
- Lower extremity—effleurage **M99.06**
- Lower extremity popliteal fossa release—MFR, BLT **M99.06**
- Abdomen—diaphragm
  - ➤ Doming technique **M99.09**
  - ➤ Thoracolumbar junction: MET, MFR, HVLA **M99.02**, **M99.03**
- Abdomen/other/viscerosomatic—Chapman's reflex for heart **M99.09**

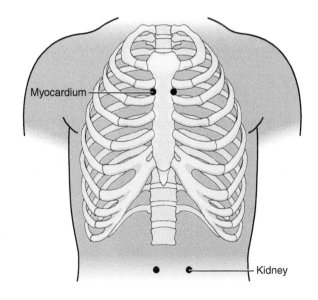

CONSTIPATION

 BASICS

DESCRIPTION

Infrequent or incomplete bowel movements

 PHYSIOLOGY AND ASSOCIATED SOMATIC DYSFUNCTIONS

PARASYMPATHETICS

- Increased tone = increased peristalsis
- Vagus nerve
  - ➤ Vagus nerve (CN X) exits the jugular foramen (composed of occiput and temporal bones).
    - → Somatic dysfunctions of occipitoatlantal joint (OA), atlantoaxial joint (AA), C2
    - → Compression of occipitomastoid sutures
- Pelvic splanchnics
  - ➤ Sacral dysfunctions
  - ➤ Innominate dysfunctions

SYMPATHETICS

- Increased tone = decreased peristalsis
- Somatic dysfunctions of T5–L2
- Superior and inferior mesenteric ganglia
  - ➤ Fascial restrictions

 OTHER SOMATIC DYSFUNCTIONS

- Thoracoabdominal diaphragm dysfunction
- Pelvic diaphragm dysfunction

TREATMENT

 2-MINUTE TREATMENT

- Sacrum—sacral articulation and distraction ART **M99.04**
- Abdomen—collateral ganglia release **M99.09**

 5-MINUTE TREATMENT

- Head—OA release **M99.00**
- Abdomen—colonic stimulation **M99.09**

 EXTENDED TREATMENT

- Cervical—AA, C2: FPR or HVLA **M99.01**
- Thoracic—MET or HVLA **M99.02**
- Rib raising **M99.08**
- Lumbar—MET or HVLA **M99.03**
- Pelvic—innominate MET **M99.05**
- Pelvic—pelvic floor muscles release: DIR **M99.06**
- Sacral dysfunctions—MET **M99.04**
- Sacrum—sacral rocking **M99.04**
- Lower extremity—iliotibial band Chapman's reflex for colon **M99.06**
- Abdomen—mesenteric lift **M99.09**
- Abdomen/other/viscerosomatic—anterior Chapman's reflex **M99.09**

C

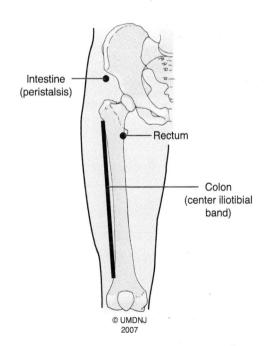

© UMDNJ
2007

COSTOCHONDRITIS

 BASICS

DESCRIPTION

Musculoskeletal chest pain along the sternal border or at the costochondral junction; may have inflammatory component; may be posttraumatic, including poststernotomy

 PHYSIOLOGY AND ASSOCIATED SOMATIC DYSFUNCTIONS

PARASYMPATHETICS

Not applicable

SYMPATHETICS

Not applicable

MOTOR

Somatic dysfunctions of C3–C5 (phrenic nerve to the diaphragm; irritation because of decreased excursion and overuse)

 OTHER SOMATIC DYSFUNCTIONS

- Rib dysfunctions
- Sternal dysfunctions
- Clavicular dysfunction
- Scalene muscle hypertonicity and tenderpoints
- Sternocleidomastoid muscle hypertonicity and tenderpoints
- Pectoralis minor muscle hypertonicity and tenderpoints
- Pectoralis major muscle hypertonicity and tenderpoints
- Serratus anterior muscle hypertonicity and tenderpoints
- Thoracic inlet diaphragm dysfunctions
- Thoracoabdominal diaphragm dysfunction
- Tenderness along the sternal border or at the costochondral junction

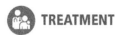 **TREATMENT**

 2-MINUTE TREATMENT

- Rib—MET **M99.08**

 5-MINUTE TREATMENT

- Sternum—BLT, MFR **M99.08**
- Thoracic—MET or HVLA **M99.02**

 EXTENDED TREATMENT

- Cervical—MFR, MET, HVLA, or FPR **M99.01**
- Cervical—scalene muscle: CS, MFR, or MET **M99.01**
- Cervical—sternocleidomastoid muscle: CS, MFR, or MET **M99.01**
- Thoracic—MFR **M99.02**
- Thoracic—thoracic inlet: BLT **M99.02**
- Thoracic—MFR **M99.02**
- Thoracolumbar—MFR, MET, or HVLA **M99.02**, **M99.03**
- Rib—BLT **M99.08**
- Upper extremity—pectoralis minor muscle: CS, MFR, or MET **M99.07**
- Upper extremity—pectoralis major muscle: CS, MFR, or MET **M99.07**
- Upper extremity—serratus anterior muscle: CS, MFR, or MET **M99.07**
- Upper extremity—clavicle: MET **M99.07**
- Abdomen diaphragm—doming technique **M99.09**

DEPRESSION

 BASICS

DESCRIPTION

A mood disorder characterized by altered emotional state, anhedonia, and altered appetite and sleep; often associated with somatic complaints and frequently comorbid with chronic illness, especially chronic pain. Gastrointestinal complaints are very common due to serotonin's effects on the gut and central nervous system.

 PHYSIOLOGY AND ASSOCIATED SOMATIC DYSFUNCTIONS

PARASYMPATHETICS

- Increased tone = decreased acid secretion, nausea, and peristalsis
- Vagus nerve
  - ➤ Somatic dysfunctions of occipitoatlantal joint (OA), atlantoaxial joint (AA), C2
- Compression of occipitomastoid sutures as well as occipitoatlantoid joint
- Pelvic splanchnic nerves
  - ➤ S2–S5—tenderpoints
    - → Sacral dysfunctions

SYMPATHETICS

- Somatic dysfunctions of T1–S2
- Celiac ganglion—fascial restriction
- Superior mesenteric ganglion—fascial restriction
- Inferior mesenteric ganglion—fascial restriction

 OTHER SOMATIC DYSFUNCTIONS

- Abdominal complaints and somatic dysfunction
- Pelvic pain and somatic dysfunction
- Compensatory changes due to poor posturing
- Look for cranial dysfunctions affecting frontal lobes (e.g., frontal compression, facial bone dysfunction).

TREATMENT

 2-MINUTE TREATMENT

- Head—OA release **M99.00**
- Rib raising **M99.08**

 5-MINUTE TREATMENT

- Cervical—ST or MFR **M99.01**
- Thoracic—ST or MFR **M99.02**
- Lumbar—ST or MFR **M99.03**

 EXTENDED TREATMENT

- Head—cranial dysfunction **M99.00**
  - Vault hold
  - CV4
- Cervical—MET, MFR, and/or HVLA **M99.01**
- Thoracic—MET, MFR, and/or HVLA **M99.02**
- Lumbar—MET, MFR, and/or HVLA **M99.03**
- Innominate—MET **M99.05**
- Sacrum—MET **M99.04**
- Abdomen/other/viscerosomatic—Chapman's reflex at ITB **M99.09**
- Abdomen/other/viscerosomatic—ganglion treatment: MFR **M99.09**

Continued

D

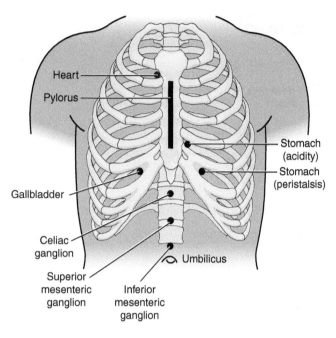

Heart
Pylorus
Stomach (acidity)
Stomach (peristalsis)
Gallbladder
Celiac ganglion
Umbilicus
Superior mesenteric ganglion
Inferior mesenteric ganglion

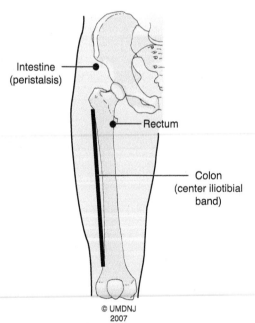

Intestine (peristalsis)
Rectum
Colon (center iliotibial band)

© UMDNJ
2007

DIARRHEA

 BASICS

DESCRIPTION

Abnormally high frequency and volume of bowel movements; may have functional, inflammatory, or infectious etiology

 PHYSIOLOGY AND ASSOCIATED SOMATIC DYSFUNCTIONS

PARASYMPATHETICS

- Increased tone = increased peristalsis
- Vagus nerve
  - ➤ Somatic dysfunctions of occipitoatlantal joint (OA), atlantoaxial joint (AA), C2, cranial and cervical dysfunction
  - ➤ Compression of occipitomastoid sutures as well as occipitoatlantoid joint
- Pelvic splanchnics S2–S4
  - ➤ Sacral dysfunction

SYMPATHETICS

- Increased tone = decreased peristalsis
- T5–L2—thoracic and lumbar dysfunction
- Celiac ganglion—fascial restriction
- Superior mesenteric ganglion—fascial restriction
- Inferior mesenteric ganglion—fascial restriction

 OTHER SOMATIC DYSFUNCTIONS

- Associated rib dysfunctions
- Thoracoabdominal diaphragm dysfunction
- Pelvic diaphragm dysfunction

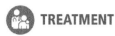 **TREATMENT**

 2-MINUTE TREATMENT

- Thoracic—ST or MFR **M99.02**
- Lumbar—ST or MFR **M99.03**

 5-MINUTE TREATMENT

- Thoracic—MET or HVLA **M99.02**
- Lumbar—MET or HVLA **M99.03**
- Abdomen—collateral ganglia release **M99.09**
- Head—OA release **M99.00**

 EXTENDED TREATMENT

- Head—V spread **M99.00**
- Cervical—FPR and/or HVLA **M99.01**
- Ribs—MET or HVLA **M99.08**
- Rib raising **M99.08**
- Sacrum—MET **M99.04**
- Innominate—MET **M99.05**
- Abdomen/other/viscerosomatic—Chapman's reflex **M99.09**

D

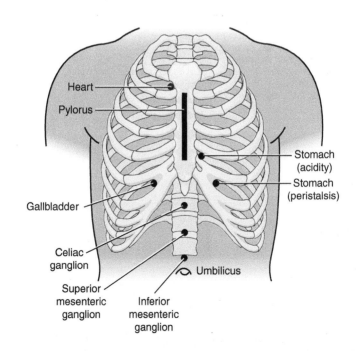

DUPUYTREN CONTRACTURE/TRIGGER FINGER

 BASICS

DESCRIPTION

Painless flexure contracture of the fingers; tendinopathy and shortening of the digital flexors with palpable and often visibly contracted tendons in the palm; may be associated with trigger fingers

 PHYSIOLOGY AND ASSOCIATED SOMATIC DYSFUNCTIONS

PARASYMPATHETICS

Not applicable

SYMPATHETICS

- Increased tone = dilated arterioles of the muscles (cholinergic and adrenergic β2), constricted arterioles of the muscles (adrenergic α)
- Somatic dysfunctions of T5–T7

MOTOR

- Median nerve (C8–T1)—flexor digitorum superficialis muscle
- Median nerve (C7–C8)—flexor digitorum profundus (second and third digits)
- Ulnar nerve (C7–T1)—flexor digitorum profundus (fourth and fifth digits)

 OTHER SOMATIC DYSFUNCTIONS

- Flexor retinaculum (transverse carpal ligament)
- Metacarpal bone somatic dysfunction
- Carpal bone somatic dysfunction
- Interosseous membrane of forearm—fascial restriction, muscle hypertonicity
- Medial epicondylitis
- Radial head dysfunction

TREATMENT

2-MINUTE TREATMENT

- Upper extremity—flexor retinaculum: MFR **M99.07**

5-MINUTE TREATMENT

- Upper extremity—interosseous membrane, forearm flexors, lumbricals and tendons in palm: BLT and MFR **M99.07**
- Thoracic—MET **M99.02**

EXTENDED TREATMENT

- Cervical—FPR, MFR, and/or HVLA **M99.01**
- Thoracic—FPR, MFR, and/or HVLA **M99.02**
- Upper extremity—carpal bone: CS, MET, and/or HVLA **M99.07**
- Upper extremity—palm/elbow/forearm treatment: CS, MFR, MET, or HVLA **M99.07**

D

DYSMENORRHEA

 BASICS

DESCRIPTION
Painful menstruation

 PHYSIOLOGY AND ASSOCIATED SOMATIC DYSFUNCTIONS

PARASYMPATHETICS

- Increased tone = uterine vasodilation
- Pelvic splanchnic nerves S2–S4—sacral dysfunction

SYMPATHETICS

- Increased tone = uterine vasoconstriction
- T10–L2—thoracic and lumbar dysfunction
- Superior mesenteric ganglion—fascial restriction
- Inferior mesenteric ganglion—fascial restriction

 OTHER SOMATIC DYSFUNCTIONS

- Restriction of ischial rectal fossa
- Pelvic diaphragm somatic dysfunction and restrictions at all attachments
- Innominate dysfunction
- Respiratory diaphragm somatic dysfunction and restrictions at all attachments

TREATMENT

 2-MINUTE TREATMENT

- Sacral base inhibition **M99.04**
- Sacral rocking **M99.04**

 5-MINUTE TREATMENT

- Sacral dysfunction—MET **M99.04**
- Innominate dysfunction—MET **M99.05**

 EXTENDED TREATMENT

D

- Innominate—ischial rectal fossa: DIR **M99.05**
- Abdomen/other—diaphragm: doming technique **M99.09**
- Thoracic—MET, soft tissue, MFR, and/or HVLA **M99.02**
- Lumbar—MET, soft tissue, MFR, and/or HVLA **M99.03**
- Abdomen/other—ganglion somatic dysfunction: MFR **M99.09**
- Abdomen/other/viscerosomatic—Chapman's reflexes for ovaries and uterus **M99.09**

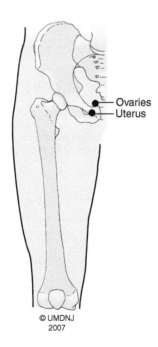

Ovaries
Uterus

© UMDNJ
2007

DYSPAREUNIA/PELVIC PAIN

 BASICS

DESCRIPTION

Pelvic pain with intercourse. Commonly, physical symptoms are accompanied by stress reactions, anxiety, or other mood disorders. Somatic dysfunctions should be suspected after trauma, birth, and surgeries; comorbid with gynecologic diagnoses (e.g., endometriosis) and gastrointestinal diagnoses (e.g., irritable bowel syndrome, inflammatory bowel disease).

 PHYSIOLOGY AND ASSOCIATED SOMATIC DYSFUNCTIONS

PARASYMPATHETICS

- Increased tone = uterine vasodilation
- Pelvic splanchnic nerves S4—sacral dysfunction

SYMPATHETICS

- Increased tone = uterine vasoconstriction
- T10–L2—thoracic and lumbar dysfunction
- Superior mesenteric ganglion—fascial restriction
- Inferior mesenteric ganglion—fascial restriction

MOTOR

- Somatic dysfunction of the sacrum (S2–S4—pudendal nerve innervates pelvic diaphragm muscles)

 OTHER SOMATIC DYSFUNCTIONS

- Pelvic diaphragm somatic dysfunction and restrictions at all attachments
- Innominate dysfunction
- Respiratory diaphragm somatic dysfunction and restrictions at all attachments
- Abdominal somatic dysfunction, including inferior mesenteric ganglion

TREATMENT

 2-MINUTE TREATMENT

- Lumbar dysfunction—MET **M99.03**
- Innominate dysfunction—MET **M99.05**
- Sacral dysfunction—MET **M99.04**

 5-MINUTE TREATMENT

- Thoracoabdominal diaphragm—doming technique **M99.09**
- Innominate—ischial rectal fossa: MFR **M99.05**

 EXTENDED TREATMENT

- Sacral rocking **M99.04**
- Thoracic—MET, soft tissue, MFR, and/or HVLA **M99.02**
- Lumbar—soft tissue, MFR, and/or HVLA **M99.03**
- Abdomen/other—ganglion restriction: MFR **M99.09**
- Abdomen/other/viscerosomatic—Chapman's reflexes if found for gastrointestinal or pelvic organs **M99.09**

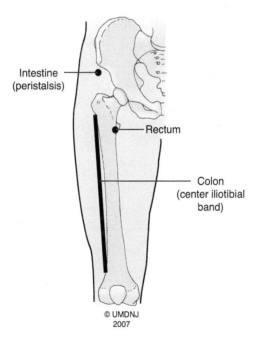

Intestine (peristalsis)

Rectum

Colon (center iliotibial band)

© UMDNJ
2007

Continued

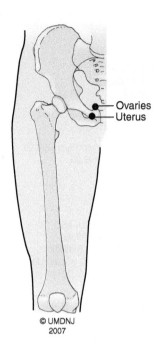

Ovaries
Uterus

© UMDNJ
2007

DYSPHAGIA

 BASICS

DESCRIPTION

Difficult and often painful swallowing

 PHYSIOLOGY AND ASSOCIATED SOMATIC DYSFUNCTIONS

PARASYMPATHETICS

- Increased tone = increased peristalsis
- Vagus nerve (CN X) exits the jugular foramen (composed of occiput and temporal bones).
  - ➤ Somatic dysfunctions of occipitoatlantal joint (OA), atlantoaxial joint (AA), C2
  - ➤ Compression of occipitomastoid sutures

SYMPATHETICS

- Increased tone = decreased peristalsis
- Somatic dysfunction of
  - ➤ T1–T4—head and neck
  - ➤ T5–T10—upper gastrointestinal tract
  - ➤ Celiac ganglion—fascial restriction

MOTOR

- Somatic dysfunction of C3–C5 (phrenic nerve to the diaphragm)
- Hypoglossal nerve (CN IX) (innervated the tongue)
  - ➤ Somatic dysfunctions of occipitoatlantal joint (OA), atlantoaxial joint (AA), C2
- Accessory nerve (CN XI) (innervated the trapezius) exits the jugular foramen (composed of occiput and temporal bones).
  - ➤ Compression of occipitomastoid sutures

 OTHER SOMATIC DYSFUNCTIONS

- Anterior cervical myofascial somatic dysfunctions
- Scapular dysfunction affecting the omohyoid muscle
- Respiratory diaphragm somatic dysfunction of motion and restriction at all attachments

TREATMENT

 2-MINUTE TREATMENT

- Head—vagus nerve: OA release **M99.00**
- Cervical—anterior cervical: MFR **M99.01**

 5-MINUTE TREATMENT

- Cervical—MET, MFR, FPR, and/or HVLA **M99.01**
- Thoracic—MFR and/or HVLA **M99.02**

 EXTENDED TREATMENT

- Head—cranial strains: vault hold **M99.00**
- Upper extremity—scapular release MFR, BLT **M99.07**
- Abdomen/other—celiac ganglion: MFR **M99.09**
- Abdomen/other—diaphragm attachments (costal margins, T12–L1, xiphoid process): MFR **M99.09**
- Abdomen/other—diaphragm doming **M99.09**
- Abdomen/other/viscerosomatic—Chapman's reflex for stomach **M99.09**

D

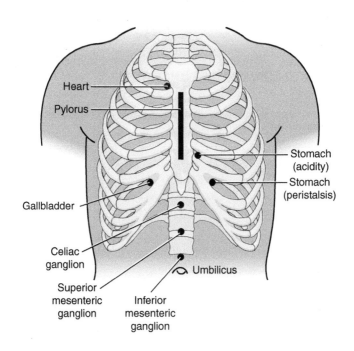

EMESIS

 BASICS

DESCRIPTION

Vomiting is a symptom of another disease process and may be associated with gastroenteritis, hyperemesis gravidarum, gastroesophageal reflux disease, cholecystitis, vertigo, and many other diagnoses.

 PHYSIOLOGY AND ASSOCIATED SOMATIC DYSFUNCTIONS

PARASYMPATHETICS

- Increased tone = increased peristalsis
- Vagus nerve
  - ➤ Vagus nerve (CN X) exits the jugular foramen (composed of occiput and temporal bones).
    - → Somatic dysfunctions of occipitoatlantal joint (OA), atlantoaxial joint (AA), C2
    - → Compression of occipitomastoid sutures

SYMPATHETICS

- Increased tone = decreased peristalsis
- Somatic dysfunctions of T5–T9
- Celiac ganglion—fascial restriction

MOTOR

- Somatic dysfunctions of C3–C5 (phrenic nerve to the diaphragm; irritation because of proximity to stomach)

 OTHER SOMATIC DYSFUNCTIONS

- Cranial dysfunctions
- Respiratory diaphragm somatic dysfunction of motion and restrictions at all attachments
- Other gastrointestinal Chapman's reflex

TREATMENT

 2-MINUTE TREATMENT

- Head—vagus nerve: OA release MFR **M99.00**
- Abdomen/other/viscerosomatic—Chapman's reflex for stomach and esophagus **M99.09**

 5-MINUTE TREATMENT

- Thoracic—MET **M99.02**
- Abdomen/other—celiac ganglion: MFR **M99.09**

 EXTENDED TREATMENT

- Cervical—C2; C3–C5: MFR, FPR, and/or HVLA **M99.01**
- Thoracic—T5–T9: MFR and/or HVLA **M99.02**
- Abdomen/other—diaphragm attachments (costal margins, T12–L1, xiphoid process): MFR **M99.09**
- Abdomen/other—diaphragm: doming MET/MFR **M99.09**

E

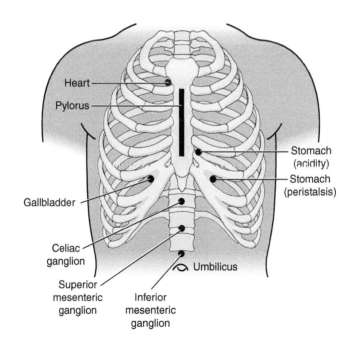

ERECTILE DYSFUNCTION

 BASICS

DESCRIPTION

A disorder usually referring to the inability to obtain and/or maintain an adequate erection for satisfactory sexual activity

 PHYSIOLOGY AND ASSOCIATED SOMATIC DYSFUNCTIONS

PARASYMPATHETICS

- Increased tone = vasodilation, erection
- Pelvic splanchnic nerves
- S2–S4—sacral dysfunction

SYMPATHETICS

- Increased tone = vasoconstriction, ejaculation
- T11–L2—thoracic and lumbar dysfunction

 OTHER SOMATIC DYSFUNCTIONS

- Restriction and muscle tension of ischial rectal fossa
- Innominate dysfunction
- Pelvic diaphragm somatic dysfunction and restriction at all attachments
- Respiratory diaphragm somatic dysfunction and restrictions at all attachments

TREATMENT

 2-MINUTE TREATMENT

- Lumbar—soft tissue or MFR **M99.03**
- Sacral rocking **M99.04**

 5-MINUTE TREATMENT

- Sacral dysfunction—MET **M99.04**
- Innominate dysfunction—MET **M99.05**

 EXTENDED TREATMENT

- Thoracic—MET, soft tissue, MFR, and/or HVLA **M99.02**
- Lumbar—MET, soft tissue, MFR, and/or HVLA **M99.03**
- Innominate—ischial rectal fossa: MFR **M99.05**
- Abdomen/other/viscerosomatic—Chapman's reflexes for prostate **M99.09**

E

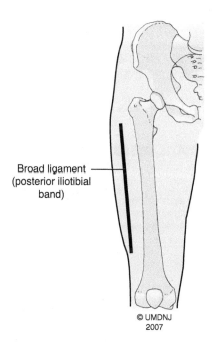

Broad ligament
(posterior iliotibial
band)

© UMDNJ
2007

FIBROMYALGIA

 BASICS

DESCRIPTION

Chronic, widespread body pain is the primary symptom. A variety of other symptoms are common including moderate to severe fatigue, sleep disorders, problems with cognitive functioning, IBS, bruxism, headaches and migraines, anxiety and depression, and environmental sensitivities.

 PHYSIOLOGY AND ASSOCIATED SOMATIC DYSFUNCTIONS

PARASYMPATHETICS

- Increased tone = bradycardia, increased acid secretion, increased peristalsis, nausea, vomiting, diarrhea
- Vagus nerve
  - ➤ Vagus nerve (CN X) exits the jugular foramen (composed of occiput and temporal bones).
  - ➤ Somatic dysfunctions of occipitoatlantal joint (OA), atlantoaxial joint (AA), C2
  - ➤ Compression of occipitomastoid sutures

SYMPATHETICS

- Increased tone = tachycardia, constipation, increased sensitivity to acid, decreased peristalsis
- Somatic dysfunction—T1–T4 and/or T5–L2
- Prevertebral ganglia
  - ➤ Celiac ganglion—fascial restriction
  - ➤ Superior mesenteric ganglion—fascial restriction
  - ➤ Inferior mesenteric ganglion—fascial restriction

MOTOR

- Somatic dysfunction C2–C7 (levator scapulae muscles, scalene muscle; irritation associated with anxiety/stress)

 OTHER SOMATIC DYSFUNCTIONS

- Cranial dysfunction
- General fascial restrictions
- TMJ dysfunction—medial and lateral pterygoid muscle hypertonicity
- Trigger points and hypertonicity of upper trapezius muscle, levator scapulae muscle, sternocleidomastoid muscle, and pectoralis muscles

TREATMENT

 2-MINUTE TREATMENT

- Head—OA release MFR **M99.00**

 5-MINUTE TREATMENT

- Cervical—FPR **M99.01**

 EXTENDED TREATMENT

- Head—cranial strain pattern **M99.00**
    - ➤ Vault hold
    - ➤ CV4 hold
- Cervical—CS, FPR, and/or MFR **M99.01**
- Thoracic— CS, FPR, and/or MFR **M99.02**
- Lumbar— CS, FPR, and/or MFR **M99.03**
- PINS technique to line segments of pain **M99.09**
- Abdomen/other/viscerosomatic—Chapman's reflex at ITB **M99.09**
- Abdomen/other/viscerosomatic—ganglion restriction: MFR **M99.09**
- Lower extremity—CS, FPR, and/or MFR **M99.06**
- Upper extremity—CS, FPR, and/or MFR **M99.07**

Continued   F

FIBROMYALGIA

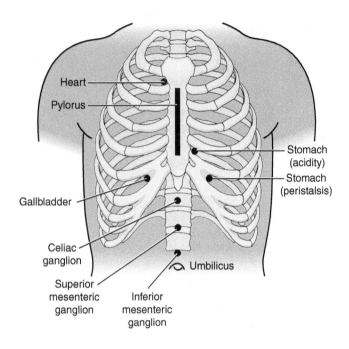

Heart
Pylorus
Stomach (acidity)
Stomach (peristalsis)
Gallbladder
Celiac ganglion
Superior mesenteric ganglion
Umbilicus
Inferior mesenteric ganglion

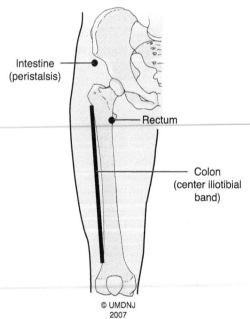

Intestine (peristalsis)
Rectum
Colon (center iliotibial band)

© UMDNJ
2007

FROZEN SHOULDER

 BASICS

DESCRIPTION

A painful limitation of motion of the shoulder resulting from chronic inflammation or posttraumatic scar tissue of the rotator cuff, also known as adhesive capsulitis

 PHYSIOLOGY AND ASSOCIATED SOMATIC DYSFUNCTIONS

PARASYMPATHETICS

Not applicable

SYMPATHETICS

- Increased tone = dilated arterioles of the muscles (cholinergic and adrenergic β2), constricted arterioles of the muscles (adrenergic α)
- Somatic dysfunctions of T1–T5

MOTOR

Primary Motion	Muscle	Innervation
Flexion	Deltoid (anterior)	Axillary nerve C5–C6
	Pectoralis major	Lateral and medial pectoral nerves; clavicular head (C5 and C6), sternocostal head (C7, C8, and T1)
Extension	Deltoid (posterior)	Axillary nerve C5–C6
	Latissimus dorsi	Thoracodorsal (long scapular) nerve C6–C8
	Teres major	Lower subscapular nerve C5–C6
Abduction	Deltoid (middle)	Axillary nerve C5–C6
	Supraspinatus	Suprascapular nerve C5–C6
Adduction	Pectoralis major (lower)	Lateral and medial pectoral nerves; clavicular head (C5 and C6), sternocostal head (C7, C8, and T1)
	Latissimus dorsi	Thoracodorsal (long scapular) nerve C6–C8
	Teres major	Lower subscapular nerve C5–C6
Internal/medial rotation	Pectoralis major	Lateral and medial pectoral nerves; clavicular head (C5 and C6), sternocostal head (C7, C8, and T1)
	Subscapularis	Upper and lower subscapular nerve C5–C6
	Latissimus dorsi	Thoracodorsal (long scapular) nerve C6–C8
	Teres major	Lower subscapular nerve C5–C6
External/lateral rotation	Infraspinatus	Suprascapular nerve C5–C6
	Teres minor	Axillary nerve C5–C6

 OTHER SOMATIC DYSFUNCTIONS

- Clavicle somatic dysfunction
- Levator scapulae muscle hypertonicity, tenderpoints, and restricted motion
- Ribs 1–9 somatic dysfunction
- Trapezius muscle hypertonicity, tenderpoints, and restricted motion
- Rhomboid major muscle and rhomboid minor muscle hypertonicity with corresponding C7–T5 dysfunction
- Pectoralis minor muscle hypertonicity, tenderpoints, and restricted motion
- Lateral and medial epicondylar tenderpoints

SPECIALIZED TESTING

- Apley's scratch test
- Drop arm test
- Neer's test
- Speed's test
- Yergason's test
- Apprehension test
- Adson's test
- Military posture test
- Wright's test

 TREATMENT

 2-MINUTE TREATMENT

- Upper extremity—Spencer technique **M99.07**

 5-MINUTE TREATMENT

- Trapezius muscle—DIR (trapezius muscle release) **M99.07**
- Thoracic—MET **M99.02**

 EXTENDED TREATMENT

- Cervical—FPR, MFR, and/or HVLA **M99.01**
- Thoracic—FPR, MFR, and/or HVLA **M99.02**
- Ribs 1 and 2—FPR, MET **M99.08**
- Upper extremity muscles—CS, MET **M99.07**
- Upper extremity—epicondyles: CS **M99.07**
- Upper extremity—clavicle: BLT, ART, MET **M99.07**

F

GASTRITIS/GASTROESOPHAGEAL REFLUX DISEASE/DYSPEPSIA

 BASICS

DESCRIPTION

Inflammation of the stomach

 PHYSIOLOGY AND ASSOCIATED SOMATIC DYSFUNCTIONS

PARASYMPATHETICS

- Increased tone = increased acid production and peristalsis
  - ➤ Vagus nerve (CN X) exits the jugular foramen (composed of occiput and temporal bones).
  - ➤ Somatic dysfunctions of occipitoatlantal joint (OA), atlantoaxial joint (AA), C2
  - ➤ Compression of occipitomastoid sutures

SYMPATHETICS

- Increased tone = decreased acid production and peristalsis
- Somatic dysfunctions of T5–T9
- Prevertebral ganglion: celiac, superior mesenteric ganglion restriction

MOTOR

- Somatic dysfunction of C3–C5 (phrenic nerve to the diaphragm; irritation caused by proximity to diaphragm)

 OTHER SOMATIC DYSFUNCTIONS

- Pterygoid spasm
- Thoracic outlet—somatic dysfunction of clavicle, first rib, scalene muscles, T1 (left thoracic duct fascial restriction)
- Diaphragm—restriction of gross motion and at all attachments
- Mesenteric restriction
- Cisterna chyli—fascial restriction

TREATMENT

 2-MINUTE TREATMENT

- Abdomen/other/viscerosomatic—celiac and superior mesenteric ganglion: MFR **M99.09**

 5-MINUTE TREATMENT

- Thoracic—seated MET **M99.02**
- Abdomen/other/viscerosomatic—Chapman's reflex for stomach **M99.09**
  ➤ Left fifth and sixth ICS near sternum

 EXTENDED TREATMENT

- Head—vagus nerve: OA release, V spread technique of occipitomastoid suture, pterygoid release DIR (to help with OA) **M99.00**
- Cervical—C2, C3–C5: MFR, FPR, and/or HVLA **M99.01**
- Thoracic—MFR and/or HVLA **M99.02**
- Abdomen/other/viscerosomatic—left thoracic duct: lymphatic **M99.09**
- Abdomen/other/viscerosomatic—cisterna chyli, fascial: lymphatic **M99.09**
- Abdomen/other—diaphragm
  ➤ Doming technique **M99.09**
  ➤ Thoracolumbar junction—MET, MFR, or HVLA **M99.02** and/or **M99.03**
- Abdomen/other—mesenteric release **M99.09**

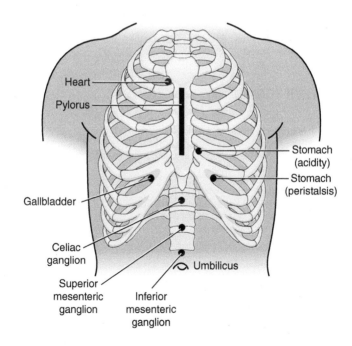

G

HEADACHE

 BASICS

DESCRIPTION

Pain in the head that is localized to the cranial vault, although it may include the region of the eyes or the back of the upper neck

 PHYSIOLOGY AND ASSOCIATED SOMATIC DYSFUNCTIONS

PARASYMPATHETICS

- Increased tone = constricts pupil; significantly increased secretions of nasal, lacrimal, and submandibular glands
- Facial nerve (CN VII), glossopharyngeal nerve (CN IX)—cranial dysfunction
- Vagus nerve (CN X) exits the jugular foramen (composed of occiput and temporal bones).
  - ➤ Somatic dysfunctions of occipitoatlantal joint (OA), atlantoaxial joint (AA), C2
  - ➤ Compression of occipitomastoid sutures

SYMPATHETICS

- Increased tone = vasoconstriction and slight secretions of nasal, lacrimal, and submandibular glands; increased blood flow to skeletal muscle
- Somatic dysfunction of T1–T5

MOTOR

- C2–C7 somatic dysfunction (levator scapulae muscle, scalene muscle; irritation associated with anxiety/stress)
- Accessory nerve (CN XI) (innervated the trapezius) exits the jugular foramen (composed of occiput and temporal bones).
  - ➤ Compression of occipitomastoid sutures

 OTHER SOMATIC DYSFUNCTIONS

- Venous sinus restrictions
- Any cranial or facial bone somatic dysfunction
- Any cervical dysfunction
- TMJ dysfunction—medial pterygoid, posterior digastric muscles, and glossal muscles; hyoid muscles; and fascial restrictions
- Trigger points
  - ➤ Trapezius muscle hypertonicity and tenderness
  - ➤ Rectus capitis posterior (major and minor) muscles
  - ➤ Levator scapulae muscle hypertonicity and tenderness
  - ➤ SCM hypertonicity and tenderness

TREATMENT

 2-MINUTE TREATMENT

- Head—vagus nerve: OA release **M99.00**
- Cervical—FPR **M99.01**

 5-MINUTE TREATMENT

- Cervical spine—MET and/or HVLA **M99.01**
- Thoracic spine—seated MET **M99.02**

 EXTENDED TREATMENT

- Head—normalize CRI: CV4 hold **M99.00**
- Head—normalize cranial motion: vault hold **M99.00**
- Head—PINS technique to head **M99.00**
- Head—TMJ: DIR pterygoid muscles and/or posterior digastric muscle **M99.00**
- Head—rectus capitus DIR **M99.00**
- Cervical—anterior and posterior cervicals, MFR **M99.01**
- Cervical—PINS technique to cervical **M99.01**
- Thoracic—MFR and/or HVLA **M99.02**
- Upper extremity—trapezius muscle DIR (trapezius muscle release), MET **M99.07**
- Upper extremity—levator scapulae muscle MET **M99.07**
- Abdomen/other/viscerosomatic—Chapman's reflex for any corresponding illness of the head (e.g., sinusitis, otitis media) **M99.09**

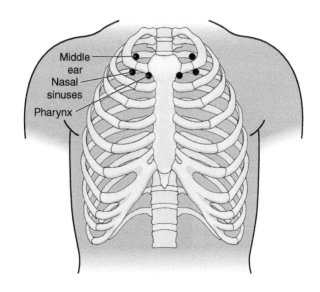

Middle ear
Nasal sinuses
Pharynx

H

HICCUPS (SINGULTUS)

 BASICS

DESCRIPTION

Spasm of the thoracoabdominal diaphragm, also known as singultus. Look for underlying cause of diaphragmatic irritation, including respiratory, gastrointestinal, and cardiac etiology.

 PHYSIOLOGY AND ASSOCIATED SOMATIC DYSFUNCTIONS

PARASYMPATHETICS

Not applicable unless comorbid organ system involved

SYMPATHETICS

Not applicable unless comorbid organ system involved

MOTOR

- C3–C5 (phrenic nerve to the diaphragm)—cervical dysfunction

 OTHER SOMATIC DYSFUNCTIONS

- Thoracoabdominal diaphragm
- Anterior scalene muscle
- Upper lumbar dysfunction (diaphragm attachment)
- Rib dysfunctions

TREATMENT

 2-MINUTE TREATMENT

- Cervical—inhibition over anterior scalene muscle (phrenic nerve) **M99.01**
- Cervical—soft tissue, MFR, FPR, and/or HVLA **M99.01**

 5-MINUTE TREATMENT

- Cervical—scalene muscles: CS and/or MET **M99.01**
- Abdominal/other—diaphragm: doming technique **M99.09**

 EXTENDED TREATMENT

- Lumbar—soft tissue, MFR, MET, or HVLA **M99.03**
- Rib dysfunction—MET **M99.08**

H

HYPERTENSION

 BASICS

DESCRIPTION

Persistently elevated blood pressure, which may be a symptom of underlying cardiac or renal disease. More often, no underlying disease process is identified (essential hypertension). The physician should look to the cardiac, renal, and autonomic nervous system for treatment options.

 PHYSIOLOGY AND ASSOCIATED SOMATIC DYSFUNCTIONS

PARASYMPATHETICS

- Increased tone = bradycardia
- Vagus nerve (CN X) exits the jugular foramen (composed of occiput and temporal bones).
  - ➤ Somatic dysfunctions of occipitoatlantal joint (OA), atlantoaxial joint (AA), C2
  - ➤ Compression of occipitomastoid sutures

SYMPATHETICS

- Increased tone = tachycardia, vasospasm
- Somatic dysfunction
  - ➤ T1–T5 cardiac
  - ➤ T10–T11 renal
- Inferior mesenteric ganglion—renal/adrenal

 OTHER SOMATIC DYSFUNCTIONS

- Lymphatic restrictions at any diaphragm and resultant edema

TREATMENT

 2-MINUTE TREATMENT

- Head—vagus nerve: OA release and/or V spread technique **M99.00**
- Rib raising **M99.08**

 5-MINUTE TREATMENT

- Thoracic—MFR, MET, and/or HVLA **M99.02**

 EXTENDED TREATMENT

- Thoracic—lymphatic pump **M99.02**
- Upper extremity, lower extremity—effleurage for lymphatic congestion **M99.07**, **M99.06**
- Abdomen/other/viscerosomatic—Chapman's reflex for heart and kidney **M99.09**
- Abdomen/other—inferior mesenteric ganglion release **M99.09**
- Abdomen/other—respiratory diaphragm release BLT and/or MET **M99.09**

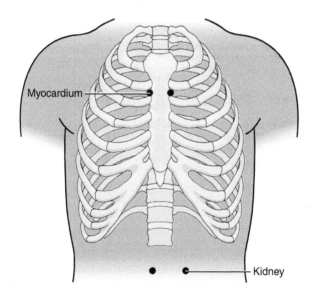

Myocardium

Kidney

H

73

ILEUS

 BASICS

DESCRIPTION

A blockage of the intestine that prevents the contents of the intestine from passing to the lower bowel, especially functional obstruction caused by absence of peristalsis

 PHYSIOLOGY AND ASSOCIATED SOMATIC DYSFUNCTIONS

PARASYMPATHETICS

- Increased tone = contracted lumen, relaxed sphincter, increased secretion and motility
- Vagus nerve (CN X) exits the jugular foramen (composed of occiput and temporal bones).
  - ➤ Somatic dysfunctions of occipitoatlantal joint (OA), atlantoaxial joint (AA), C2
  - ➤ Compression of occipitomastoid sutures
  - ➤ Pelvic splanchnics—S2–S4
- Sacroiliac dysfunctions/sacral torsions

SYMPATHETICS

- Increased tone = relaxed lumen, contracted sphincter, decreased secretions and motility
- Somatic dysfunction of T10–L4
- Prevertebral ganglion restriction
  - ➤ Celiac ganglion—fascial restriction
  - ➤ Inferior mesenteric ganglion—fascial restriction
  - ➤ Superior mesenteric ganglion—fascial restriction

 OTHER SOMATIC DYSFUNCTIONS

- Mesenteric restrictions
- Respiratory diaphragm somatic dysfunction and restriction at all attachments
- Cisterna chyli—fascial restriction
- Left thoracic duct restriction

TREATMENT

 ## 2-MINUTE TREATMENT

- Rib raising **M99.08**

 ## 5-MINUTE TREATMENT

- Sacrum—sacral rocking **M99.04**
- Abdomen/other—**M99.09**
  - ➤ Superior mesenteric ganglion: MFR
  - ➤ Mesenteric release—lymph

 ## EXTENDED TREATMENT

- Head—vagus nerve: OA release, V spread technique of occipitomastoid suture **M99.00**
- Cervical—MFR, FPR, and/or HVLA **M99.01**
- Thoracic—MFR and/or MET **M99.02**
- Abdomen/other—left thoracic duct: lymphatic **M99.09**
- Abdomen/other—cisterna chyli: facial/lymphatic **M99.09**
- Abdomen/other—respiratory diaphragm
  - ➤ Doming technique **M99.09**
  - ➤ Thoracolumbar junction—MET, MFR, HVLA **M99.02**, **M99.03**
- Abdomen/other/viscerosomatic—Chapman's reflex for intestine, colon, and rectum **M99.09**
- Abdomen/other/viscerosomatic—colonic stimulation **M99.09**
- Lower extremity—pedal pump **M99.06**

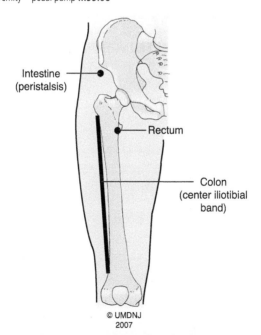

© UMDNJ
2007

INFLAMMATORY BOWEL DISEASE (CROHN'S DISEASE OR ULCERATIVE COLITIS)

 BASICS

DESCRIPTION

Disease of the gastrointestinal system characterized by abdominal pain, fever, bloating, cramping, and bloody diarrhea. Recurrent low back pain is common in these individuals. Somatic dysfunction may be a clue to inflammatory bowel disease and trigger the proper workup.

 PHYSIOLOGY AND ASSOCIATED SOMATIC DYSFUNCTIONS

PARASYMPATHETICS

- Increased tone = increased peristalsis
- Vagus nerve (CN X) exits the jugular foramen (composed of occiput and temporal bones).
  - ➤ Somatic dysfunctions of occipitoatlantal joint (OA), atlantoaxial joint (AA), C2
  - ➤ Compression of occipitomastoid sutures
- Pelvic splanchnics—S2–S4
  - ➤ Sacroiliac dysfunctions

SYMPATHETICS

- Increased tone = decreased peristalsis
- Somatic dysfunction of T5–L2
- Abdominal fascial restrictions
- Prevertebral ganglion—fascial restriction
  - ➤ Superior mesenteric ganglion—fascial restriction
  - ➤ Inferior mesenteric ganglion—fascial restriction

 OTHER SOMATIC DYSFUNCTIONS

- Rib dysfunctions
- Respiratory diaphragm somatic dysfunction
- Pelvic diaphragm somatic dysfunction
- Innominate dysfunctions

TREATMENT

 2-MINUTE TREATMENT

- Thoracic—MFR **M99.02**
- Lumbar—MFR **M99.03**

 5-MINUTE TREATMENT

- Head—OA release **M99.00**
- Thoracic—MET or HVLA **M99.02**
- Lumbar—MET or HVLA **M99.03**

 EXTENDED TREATMENT

- Head—V spread technique **M99.00**
- Cervical—AA, C2, FPR, and/or HVLA **M99.01**
- Rib raising **M99.08**
- Abdomen—collateral ganglia release **M99.09**
- Abdomen/other/viscerosomatic—Chapman's reflexes **M99.09**
- Abdomen/other/viscerosomatic—mesenteric release **M99.09**
- Innominate—MET **M99.05**
- Innominate—pelvic floor release DIR **M99.05**
- Sacrum—MET **M99.04**
- Sacrum—presacral fascia release technique **M99.04**

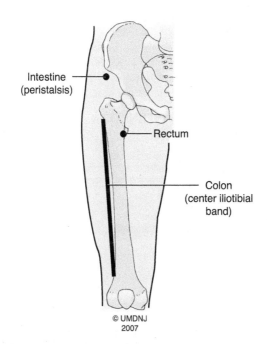

Intestine (peristalsis)

Rectum

Colon (center iliotibial band)

© UMDNJ
2007

INFLUENZA

 BASICS

DESCRIPTION

Acute, self-limited infection caused by orthomyxovirus influenza types A and B marked by inflammation of nasal mucosa, pharynx, conjunctiva, and respiratory tract passages causing fever and severe aching

 PHYSIOLOGY AND ASSOCIATED SOMATIC DYSFUNCTIONS

PARASYMPATHETICS

- Increased tone = significantly increased secretions of nasal, lacrimal, and submandibular glands
  - ➤ Facial nerve (CN VII), glossopharyngeal nerve (CN IX)—cranial dysfunction
  - ➤ Increased volume of secretions and relative bronchiole constriction
  - ➤ Vagus nerve (CN X) exits the jugular foramen (composed of occiput and temporal bones).
    - → Somatic dysfunctions of occipitoatlantal joint (OA), atlantoaxial joint (AA), C2
    - → Compression of occipitomastoid sutures
  - ➤ Vasodilation, decreased headache and facial pain
  - ➤ SPG

SYMPATHETICS

- Increased tone
  - ➤ Vasoconstriction and slight secretions of nasal, lacrimal, and submandibular glands; increased blood flow to skeletal muscle
  - ➤ Decreased secretions and bronchiole dilation
- Somatic dysfunctions of T1–T7

MOTOR

- Somatic dysfunctions of C3–C5 (phrenic nerve to the diaphragm; dysfunction as a result of decreased excursion and overuse)

 OTHER SOMATIC DYSFUNCTIONS

- Cranial and facial bone dysfunctions
- Anterior cervical and sternal fascia fascial restrictions
- Scalene muscles—hypertonicity and tenderpoints
- Sternocleidomastoid muscle—hypertonicity and tenderpoints
- Inhalation or exhalation rib dysfunctions
- Serratus anterior muscle restrictions
- Respiratory diaphragm somatic dysfunctions
- Thoracolumbar dysfunction (diaphragm attachment)

TREATMENT

 ## 2-MINUTE TREATMENT

- Rib raising **M99.08**

 ## 5-MINUTE TREATMENT

- Thoracic—MET and/or HVLA **M99.02**

 ## EXTENDED TREATMENT

- Head—decreased CRI: CV4 hold, cranial strains OCMM **M99.00**
- Head—vagus nerve: OA release **M99.00**
- Head—SPG stimulation **M99.00**
- Cervical—C2, C3–C5: MFR, FPR, and/or HVLA **M99.01**
- Cervical—scalene muscles: CS and/or MET **M99.01**
- Cervical—anterior cervical fascial release MFR **M99.01**
- Thoracic—MFR **M99.02**
- Thoracic pump—lymph **M99.02**
- Thoracolumbar junction: MET, MFR, HVLA **M99.02**, **M99.03**
- Rib dysfunction—MET **M99.08**
- Upper extremity—pectoralis minor muscle: serratus anterior muscle CS, MFR, and/or pectoralis muscle traction (for lymphatic treatment) **M99.07**
- Abdomen—doming of the diaphragm technique **M99.09**
- Abdomen/other/viscerosomatic—Chapman's reflex for lung **M99.09**
- Abdomen/other/viscerosomatic—pedal pump: **M99.09**

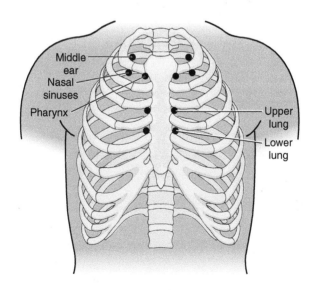

IRRITABLE BOWEL SYNDROME

 BASICS

DESCRIPTION

Disease of the gastrointestinal system characterized by abdominal pain, bloating, cramping, and mixed predominance of diarrhea or constipation often associated with stress, depression, and anxiety

 PHYSIOLOGY AND ASSOCIATED SOMATIC DYSFUNCTIONS

PARASYMPATHETICS

- Increased tone = decreased heart rate, increased peristalsis, nausea, vomiting, bowel
- Vagus nerve (CN X) exits the jugular foramen (composed of occiput and temporal bones).
  - Somatic dysfunctions of occipitoatlantal joint (OA), atlantoaxial joint (AA), C2
  - Compression of occipitomastoid sutures
- Pelvic splanchnic nerves—S2–S4
  - Sacral and innominate dysfunctions

SYMPATHETICS

- Increased tone = tachycardia, increased sensitivity to acid, decreased bowel motility/ constipation
- Somatic dysfunctions
  - T1–T4 (cardiac) and/or T5–L2 (gastrointestinal) decreased peristalsis
- Prevertebral ganglion—fascial restriction
  - Celiac ganglion—fascial restriction
  - Superior mesenteric ganglion—fascial restriction
  - Inferior mesenteric ganglion—fascial restriction

 OTHER SOMATIC DYSFUNCTIONS

- Rib dysfunctions
- Respiratory diaphragm somatic dysfunction
- Abdominal fascial restrictions
- Pelvic diaphragm somatic dysfunction

TREATMENT

 2-MINUTE TREATMENT

- Thoracic—MET **M99.02**
- Lumbar—MET **M99.03**

 5-MINUTE TREATMENT

- Head—OA release **M99.00**
- Abdomen/other—collateral ganglia release **M99.09**

 EXTENDED TREATMENT

- Head—medial and lateral pterygoid muscles hypertonicity (TMJ) **M99.00**
- Head—V spread technique **M99.00**
- Cervical—FPR and/or HVLA **M99.01**
- Thoracic—MFR and/or HVLA **M99.02**
- Rib raising **M99.08**
- Ribs—MET **M99.08**
- Upper extremity—trigger points and hypertonicity of trapezius muscle, levator scapulae muscle, and pectoralis muscles **M99.07**
- Lumbar—MFR and/or HVLA **M99.03**
- Sacral rocking technique **M99.04**
- Sacrum—MET **M99.04**
- Innominates—MET **M99.05**
- Innominates—ischial rectal fossa release **M99.05**
- Abdomen/other/viscerosomatic—Chapman's reflex for gastrointestinal system **M99.09**

Continued

IRRITABLE BOWEL SYNDROME

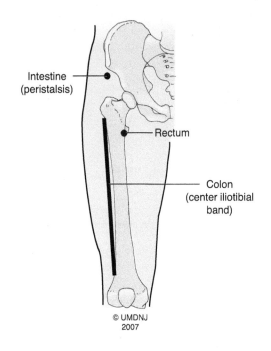

Intestine (peristalsis)

Rectum

Colon (center iliotibial band)

© UMDNJ 2007

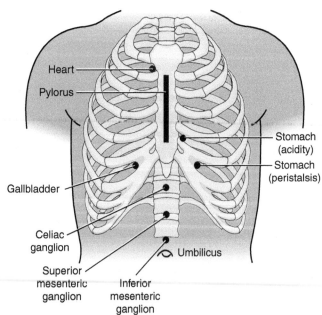

Heart

Pylorus

Stomach (acidity)

Stomach (peristalsis)

Gallbladder

Celiac ganglion

Umbilicus

Superior mesenteric ganglion

Inferior mesenteric ganglion

LATERAL EPICONDYLITIS

 BASICS

DESCRIPTION

Lateral epicondylitis (tennis elbow) is a painful inflammatory condition of the musculature attachments of the extensors of the hand and wrist as well as the supinator muscle.

 PHYSIOLOGY AND ASSOCIATED SOMATIC DYSFUNCTIONS

PARASYMPATHETICS

Not applicable

SYMPATHETICS

- Increased tone = dilated arterioles of the muscles (cholinergic and adrenergic β2), constricted arterioles of the muscles (adrenergic α)
- T1–T5—thoracic dysfunction

MOTOR

- Lateral epicondyle
  - Radial nerve—(C7–C8) extensor carpi radialis brevis muscle, (C7–C8) extensor digitorum muscle, (C7–C8) extensor digiti minimi muscle, (C6–C7) supinator muscle
    - Muscle tenderpoints and hypertonicity

 OTHER SOMATIC DYSFUNCTIONS

- Interosseous membrane of forearm fascial restriction
- Elbow somatic dysfunctions

SPECIALIZED TESTING

- Tinel's sign at elbow (ulnar nerve entrapment)
- Tennis elbow test—Mill's (epicondilitis)
- Cozen's test
- Golfer's elbow test
- Tests for ligamentous stability at elbow

 TREATMENT

 2-MINUTE TREATMENT

- Upper extremity—interosseous membrane and forearm extensors: MFR **M99.07**

 5-MINUTE TREATMENT

- Upper extremity—elbow/forearm supination dysfunctions, radial head dysfunctions: MET, HVLA **M99.07**
- Cervical—FPR, soft tissue, MFR, and/or HVLA **M99.01**

 EXTENDED TREATMENT

- Thoracic—MET, FPR, soft tissue, MFR, and/or HVLA **M99.02**
- Upper extremity—strain-counterstrain to tenderpoints found in forearm **M99.07**

LOW BACK PAIN

 BASICS

DESCRIPTION

Low back pain (LBP) is a symptom with a large variety of qualities, associated symptoms and range of causes most commonly mechanical in origin. A thorough history and physical exam including "red flag" symptoms and signs, neurological and orthopedic exam are used to rule out emergent causes of LBP and stratify treatment. Acute LBP usually resolves within 6 weeks responding to conservative treatment. Symptoms lasting more than 6 weeks are considered chronic and warrant further workup. Somatic dysfunction may be the primary cause of LBP or secondary to viscero-somatic, somato-somatic, or referred causes. In most cases imaging is not necessary.

 PHYSIOLOGY AND ASSOCIATED SOMATIC DYSFUNCTIONS

PARASYMPATHETICS

- Increased tone = increased peristalsis, gallbladder wall contraction, contracted detrusor muscle of the bladder
- Vagus nerve (CN X) exits the jugular foramen (composed of occiput and temporal bones).
  - ➤ Somatic dysfunctions of occipitoatlantal joint (OA), atlantoaxial joint (AA), C2
  - ➤ Compression of occipitomastoid sutures
- Pelvic splanchnics—S2–S4: sacroiliac dysfunctions

SYMPATHETICS

- Increased tone = decreased kidney output, decreased peristalsis, gallbladder wall relaxation, relaxed detrusor muscle of the bladder, dilated arterioles of the muscles (cholinergic and adrenergic β2), constricted arterioles of the muscles (adrenergic α)
- Somatic dysfunctions of T10–L2
- Prevertebral ganglion—fascial restriction
  - ➤ Celiac ganglion—fascial restriction
  - ➤ Superior mesenteric ganglion—fascial restriction
  - ➤ Inferior mesenteric ganglion—fascial restriction

MOTOR

Extensor	Erector spinae muscle	Segmental innervation C1–S5
	Transversospinal muscles (unilateral contraction of semispinalis, multifidus, and rotatores lumborum muscles)	Intercostal nerves 7–11; subcostal, iliohypogastric, and ilioinguinal nerves
Flexors	Abdominal wall (extrinsic: rectus abdominis, external abdominal oblique, internal abdominal obliques, and the transversus abdominis)	Intercostal nerves 7–11; subcostal, iliohypogastric, and ilioinguinal nerves
	Iliopsoas	Branches of the ventral primary rami of spinal nerves L2–L4; branches of the femoral nerve
	Quadratus lumborum muscle (pure sidebending)	Subcostal nerve L1–L4
Lateral flexors (sidebending)	Abdominal muscles (unilateral contraction as above)	Intercostal nerves 7–11; subcostal, iliohypogastric, and ilioinguinal nerves
Rotators	Transversospinal muscles (unilateral contraction as above)	Intercostal nerves 7–11; subcostal, iliohypogastric, and ilioinguinal nerves
	Abdominal muscles (unilateral contraction as above)	Intercostal nerves 7–11; subcostal, iliohypogastric, and ilioinguinal nerves

OTHER SOMATIC DYSFUNCTIONS

Hypertonicity and tenderness of associated muscles
- Adductor muscles
- Hamstring muscle
- Gluteus maximus and medius muscles
- Piriformis

 ## SPECIALIZED TESTING

- FABERE (Patrick's) test
- Leg raising
- Lumbosacral spring test
- Standing/seated flexion tests
- Thomas's test
- Trendelenburg's test

 ## TREATMENT

 2-MINUTE TREATMENT

- Lumbar spine—MET **M99.03**
- Lower extremity—psoas muscle: CS **M99.06**

 5-MINUTE TREATMENT

- Innominate dysfunction—MET **M99.05**
- Sacral dysfunction—MET **M99.04**

 EXTENDED TREATMENT

- Thoracic—MET, MFR, and/or HVLA **M99.02**
- Lumbar—MET, MFR, and/or HVLA **M99.03**
- Sacral distraction **M99.04**
- Lower extremity—muscle hypertonicity and tenderness MFR, MET, CS **M99.06**
- Abdomen/other—diaphragm: doming technique **M99.09**
- Abdomen/other—ganglion restriction: MFR **M99.09**
- Abdomen/other/viscerosomatic—Chapman's reflexes for corresponding visceral dysfunctions **M99.09**

Continued

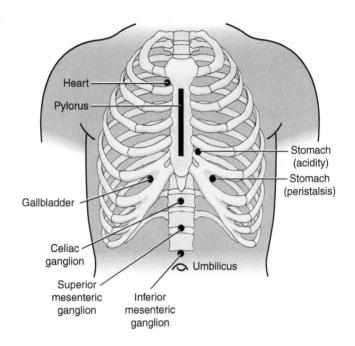

Heart

Pylorus

Stomach (acidity)

Stomach (peristalsis)

Gallbladder

Celiac ganglion

Umbilicus

Superior mesenteric ganglion

Inferior mesenteric ganglion

MEDIAL EPICONDYLITIS

 BASICS

DESCRIPTION

Medial epicondylitis (golfer's elbow) is a painful inflammatory condition of the musculature attachments of the superficial flexors of the hand and wrist as well as pronator teres muscle.

 PHYSIOLOGY AND ASSOCIATED SOMATIC DYSFUNCTIONS

PARASYMPATHETICS

Not applicable

SYMPATHETICS

- Increased tone = dilated arterioles of the muscles (cholinergic and adrenergic β2), constricted arterioles of the muscles (adrenergic α)
- T1–T5—thoracic dysfunction

MOTOR

- Medial epicondyle
  - ➤ Median nerve—(C6–C7) pronator teres muscle, (C8–T1) flexor digitorum superficialis muscle, (C7–C8) palmaris longus muscle
  - ➤ Ulnar nerve (C7–T1)—flexor carpi ulnaris muscle
    - → Muscle tenderpoints and hypertonicity

 OTHER SOMATIC DYSFUNCTIONS

- Interosseous membrane of forearm fascial restriction
- Elbow somatic dysfunctions

SPECIALIZED TESTING

- Tinel's sign at elbow (ulnar nerve entrapment)
- Tennis elbow test—Mill's (epicondilitis)
- Cozen's test
- Golfer's elbow test
- Tests for ligamentous stability at elbow

 TREATMENT

M

 2-MINUTE TREATMENT

- Upper extremity—interosseous membrane and forearm flexors: MFR **M99.07**

 5-MINUTE TREATMENT

- Upper extremity—elbow/forearm pronation dysfunctions, ulnar dysfunctions: MET, HVLA **M99.07**
- Cervical—FPR, soft tissue, MFR, and/or HVLA **M99.01**

 EXTENDED TREATMENT

- Thoracic—MET, FPR, soft tissue, MFR, and/or HVLA **M99.02**
- Upper extremity—strain-counterstrain to tenderpoints found in forearm **M99.07**

OTITIS MEDIA/SEROUS/INFECTIOUS

 BASICS

DESCRIPTION

Inflammation of the middle ear, usually associated with a viral or bacterial infection

 PHYSIOLOGY AND ASSOCIATED SOMATIC DYSFUNCTIONS

PARASYMPATHETICS

- Increased tone = copious secretions of nasal, lacrimal, and submandibular glands
- Facial nerve (CN VII)—cranial dysfunction

SYMPATHETICS

- Increased tone = vasoconstriction and slight secretions of nasal, lacrimal, and submandibular glands
- T1–T5—thoracic dysfunction (originate in thoracic spine and return to head and neck through cervical ganglia)

MOTOR

- Tensor veli palatini—CN V3
- Tensor tympani muscle—medial pterygoid branch of the CN V3
- Levator veli palatini—CN X
- Salpingopharyngeus—CN X
  - ➤ OA, AA, C2—cranial and cervical dysfunction
  - ➤ Compression of occipitomastoid sutures as well as occipitoatlantoid joint

 OTHER SOMATIC DYSFUNCTIONS

- Eustachian tube dysfunction
- Digastric muscles tenderpoints and hypertonicity
- Cranial dysfunction
- Lymphatic congestion of lymph nodes: preauricular and postauricular, submaxillary and submental, supraclavicular

TREATMENT

 2-MINUTE TREATMENT

- Head—Muncie technique **M99.00**
- Head—periauricular drainage technique **M99.00**

 5-MINUTE TREATMENT

- Head—supraorbital and infraorbital effleurage **M99.00**
- Head—sphenopalatine ganglion stimulation **M99.00**
- Cervical—soft tissue, MFR, FPR, and/or HVLA **M99.01**

 EXTENDED TREATMENT

- Head—nasion gapping **M99.00**
- Head—Galbreath technique (mandibular drainage) **M99.00**
- Head—decreased CRI: CV4 hold **M99.00**
- Head—digastric muscle: CS and/or MFR **M99.00**
- Head—vagus nerve: OA release **M99.00**
- Abdomen/other/viscerosomatic—Chapman's reflex for ear and/or sinuses **M99.09**

O

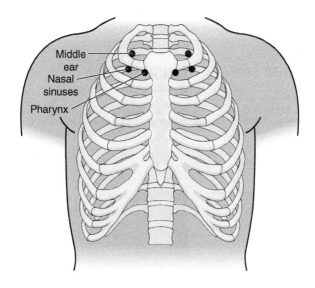

PELVIC INFLAMMATORY DISEASE

 BASICS

DESCRIPTION

Refers to infection and inflammation of the upper genital tract in women that can affect the uterus, fallopian tubes, ovaries, and other organs related to reproduction. The scarring that results on these organs can lead to infertility, ectopic pregnancy, chronic pelvic pain, abscesses, and other serious problems.

 PHYSIOLOGY AND ASSOCIATED SOMATIC DYSFUNCTIONS

PARASYMPATHETICS

- Increased tone = uterine body relaxation, constriction of the cervix, vasodilation
- Pelvic splanchnic nerves
- S2–S4—sacral dysfunction

SYMPATHETICS

- Increased tone = constriction of uterine body, relaxation of the cervix, vasoconstriction
- T12–L2—thoracic and lumbar dysfunction
- Superior mesenteric ganglion—fascial restriction
- Inferior mesenteric ganglion—fascial restriction

MOTOR

- S3–S4—sacral dysfunction, pelvic diaphragm somatic dysfunction and restriction at all attachments

 OTHER SOMATIC DYSFUNCTIONS

- Fascial restriction of ischial rectal fossa
- Innominate dysfunction
- Respiratory diaphragm somatic dysfunction and restriction at all attachments

TREATMENT

 2-MINUTE TREATMENT

- Ischial rectal fossa: MFR **M99.09**

 5-MINUTE TREATMENT

- Sacral base inhibition **M99.04**
- Innominate dysfunction—MET **M99.05**

 EXTENDED TREATMENT

- Sacral dysfunction—MET **M99.04**
- Abdomen/other—diaphragm: doming technique **M99.09**
- Thoracic—MET, soft tissue, MFR, and/or HVLA **M99.02**
- Lumbar—MET, soft tissue, MFR, and/or HVLA **M99.03**
- Abdomen/other—ganglion restriction: MFR **M99.09**
- Abdomen/other/viscerosomatic—Chapman's reflexes for ovaries and uterus **M99.09**

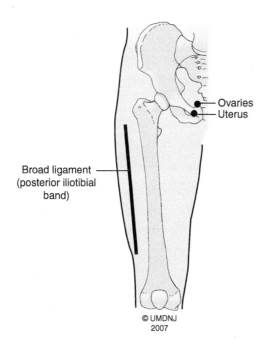

Ovaries
Uterus

Broad ligament
(posterior iliotibial
band)

© UMDNJ
2007

P

PEPTIC ULCER DISEASE

 BASICS

DESCRIPTION

A disorder characterized by hyperacidity leading to ulcers of the esophagus, stomach, and/or the duodenum

 PHYSIOLOGY AND ASSOCIATED SOMATIC DYSFUNCTIONS

PARASYMPATHETICS

● Increased tone = increased acid secretion and increased peristalsis
● Vagus nerve (CN X) exits the jugular foramen (composed of occiput and temporal bones).
  ➤ Somatic dysfunctions of occipitoatlantal joint (OA), atlantoaxial joint (AA), C2
  ➤ Compression of occipitomastoid sutures

SYMPATHETICS

● Increased tone = decreased peristalsis and decreased acid secretion
● Somatic dysfunction of T5–T10—tenderpoints
● Celiac ganglion—fascial restriction

MOTOR

● Somatic dysfunction of C3–C5 (phrenic nerve to the diaphragm; irritation caused by proximity to stomach)

 OTHER SOMATIC DYSFUNCTIONS

● Respiratory diaphragm somatic dysfunction and restriction at all attachments

TREATMENT

 ### 2-MINUTE TREATMENT

- Head—vagus nerve: OA release **M99.00**
- Abdomen/other—celiac ganglion: MFR **M99.09**

 ### 5-MINUTE TREATMENT

- Abdomen/other—respiratory diaphragm release (BLT or MET) **M99.09**
- Thoracic—MET **M99.02**

 ### EXTENDED TREATMENT

- Cervical—MFR, FPR, or HVLA **M99.01**
- Thoracic—MFR or HVLA **M99.02**
- Rib raising **M99.08**
- Abdomen/other/viscerosomatic—Chapman's reflex for stomach and esophagus **M99.09**

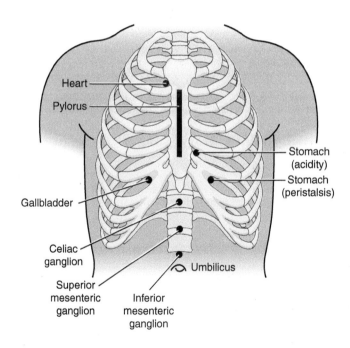

PHARYNGITIS/TONSILLITIS

 BASICS

DESCRIPTION

Infection (viral, bacterial, or fungal) of the pharynx and/or tonsils

 PHYSIOLOGY AND ASSOCIATED SOMATIC DYSFUNCTIONS

PARASYMPATHETICS

- Trigeminal nerve (CN V)
- Facial nerve (CN VII) via sphenopalatine ganglion
- Vagus nerve
  - Somatic dysfunctions of occipitoatlantal joint (OA), atlantoaxial joint (AA), C2—cranial and cervical dysfunction
  - Compression of occipitomastoid sutures as well as OA joint

SYMPATHETICS

- Somatic dysfunctions of T1–T4

MOTOR

- Trigeminal nerve (maxillary branch [CN V2]) via pharyngeal branch of pterygopalatine ganglion, superior alveolar nerves, and greater and lesser palatine nerves
- Facial nerve (CN VII) (nervus intermedius) via greater petrosal nerve and pterygopalatine ganglion
- Glossopharyngeal nerve (CN IX) via pharyngeal plexus and tonsillar and lingual branches
- Vagus nerve (CN X) via internal branch of superior laryngeal nerve and pharyngeal plexus

 OTHER SOMATIC DYSFUNCTIONS

- Eustachian tube dysfunction
- Cranial dysfunction
- Lymphatic congestion of lymph nodes: preauricular and postauricular, submaxillary and submental, supraclavicular, and anterior cervical chain

TREATMENT

 2-MINUTE TREATMENT

- Cervical—lymphatic drainage of anterior cervical lymphatic nodes/vessels **M99.01**

 5-MINUTE TREATMENT

- Head—periauricular drainage technique **M99.00**
- Abdomen/other/viscerosomatic—Chapman's reflex for pharynx just inferior to sternoclavicular joint **M99.09**
- Thoracic inlet release MFR **M99.02**

 EXTENDED TREATMENT

- Head—OA release **M99.00**
- Head—sphenopalatine ganglion stimulation **M99.00**
- Head, cervical—OA, AA, C2: soft tissue, MFR, FPR, and/or HVLA **M99.00**, **M99.01**
- Thoracic—MET, soft tissue, MFR, and/or HVLA **M99.02**
- Rib raising **M99.08**

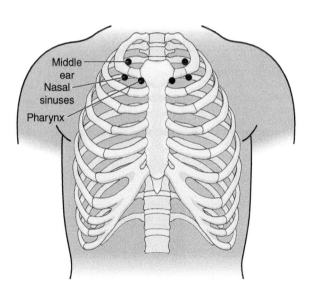

Middle
ear
Nasal
sinuses
Pharynx

P

PNEUMONIA

 BASICS

DESCRIPTION

An infectious illness of the lungs and lower respiratory system in which the alveoli become inflamed and flooded with fluid

 PHYSIOLOGY AND ASSOCIATED SOMATIC DYSFUNCTIONS

PARASYMPATHETICS

- Increased tone = thinning of secretions and relative bronchiole constriction
- Vagus nerve
  - ➤ Somatic dysfunctions of occipitoatlantal joint (OA), atlantoaxial joint (AA), C2
  - ➤ Compression of occipitomastoid sutures as well as OA joint

SYMPATHETICS

- Increased tone = thickened secretions and bronchiole dilation
- Somatic dysfunctions of T2–T7

MOTOR

- Somatic dysfunction of C3–C5 (phrenic nerve to the diaphragm; irritation caused by decreased excursion and overuse)

 OTHER SOMATIC DYSFUNCTIONS

- Scalene muscle hypertonicity and tenderpoints
- Pectoralis minor muscle hypertonicity and tenderpoints
- Serratus anterior muscle hypertonicity and tenderpoints
- Thoracic inlet myofascial restrictions
- Rib dysfunction
- Respiratory diaphragm restriction and restrictions at all attachments

TREATMENT

 2-MINUTE TREATMENT

- Thoracic pump lymphatic technique **M99.08**
- Rib raising **M99.08**

 5-MINUTE TREATMENT

- Abdomen/other—diaphragm
  - ➤ Cervical—C2, C3–C5: MFR, MET, and/or FPR **M99.01**
  - ➤ Doming technique **M99.09**
  - ➤ Thoracic inlet release—MFR **M99.02**, **M99.08**
  - ➤ Thoracolumbar junction—soft tissue, MET, MFR, HVLA **M99.02**, **M99.03**

 EXTENDED TREATMENT

- Upper extremity—pectoralis minor muscle/serratus anterior muscle: CS, soft tissue, and/or MFR **M99.07**
- Rib dysfunction—MET **M99.08**
- Cervical—scalene muscle: CS and/or MET **M99.01**
- Head—vagus nerve: OA release and/or V spread **M99.00**
- Abdomen/other/viscerosomatic—Chapman's reflex for lung **M99.09**

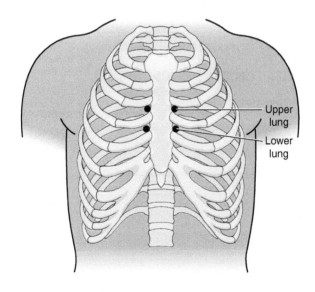

Upper lung

Lower lung

POSTCONCUSSIVE SYNDROME

 BASICS

DESCRIPTION

A form of traumatic brain injury with symptoms that include, but are not limited to, tinnitus, dizziness, headache, nausea, vomiting, depression, and cognitive impairment

 PHYSIOLOGY AND ASSOCIATED SOMATIC DYSFUNCTIONS

PARASYMPATHETICS

- Increased tone = constricts pupils; significantly increased secretions of nasal, lacrimal, and submandibular glands
- Facial nerve (CN VII), glossopharyngeal nerve (CN IX)—cranial dysfunction
- Vagus nerve
  ➤ Somatic dysfunctions of occipitoatlantal joint (OA), atlantoaxial joint (AA), C2
  ➤ Compression of occipitomastoid sutures as well as OA joint

SYMPATHETICS

- Increased tone = vasoconstriction and slight secretions of nasal, lacrimal, and submandibular glands, increased blood flow to skeletal muscle
- Somatic dysfunctions of T1–T5

MOTOR

- Oculomotor nerve (CN III), trochlear nerve (CN IV), abducens nerve (CN VI), spinal accessory nerve (CN XI), hypoglossal nerve (CN XII), C1–C8 nerve root—extraocular muscles, lingual muscles, levator scapulae muscle, longus capitis muscle, longus colli muscle, scalene muscles, splenius muscle, sternocleidomastoid muscle, rectus capitis muscle

 OTHER SOMATIC DYSFUNCTIONS

- Any cervical dysfunction
- TMJ dysfunction—medial pterygoid muscle, posterior digastric muscles, glossal muscles, hyoid muscles, and fascial restrictions

TREATMENT

 2-MINUTE TREATMENT

- Head—vagus nerve: OA release **M99.00**
- Cervical—FPR **M99.01**

 5-MINUTE TREATMENT

- Head—assess and treat CRI: CV4 **M99.00**

 EXTENDED TREATMENT

- Cervical—soft tissue, MFR, MET, and/or HVLA **M99.01**
- Thoracic—soft tissue, MFR, and/or HVLA **M99.02**
- Head—temporomandibular joint: direct inhibition to medial pterygoid muscle, genioglossal, and/or posterior digastric muscle **M99.00**
- Cervical—anterior cervical muscles and soft tissue: MFR **M99.01**
- Head—compressed cranial sutures: V spread **M99.00**
- Head—cranial strain: vault hold and/or other cranial technique **M99.00**

P

PREGNANCY

BASICS

DESCRIPTION

The duration between conception and the end of gestation. Each trimester may manifest different presentations due to rapid hormonal and biomechanical changes in the gravid mother; commonly, headaches, nausea, spinal pain, and sciatic nerve symptoms.

PHYSIOLOGY AND ASSOCIATED SOMATIC DYSFUNCTIONS

PARASYMPATHETICS

- Increased tone = increased peristalsis
- Vagus nerve
  - ➤ Somatic dysfunctions of occipitoatlantal joint (OA), atlantoaxial joint (AA), C2
- Increased tone = uterine body relaxation, constriction of the cervix
- Pelvic splanchnic nerves
- S2–S4 somatic dysfunctions
  - ➤ Sacral torsions
  - ➤ Decreased sacral motion
  - ➤ Sacroiliac joint pain

SYMPATHETICS

- Increased tone = constriction of uterine body, relaxation of the cervix
- Somatic dysfunctions of T12–L2

MOTOR

- Psoas muscle—L1–L4 somatic dysfunctions
- Piriformis—S1–S2 somatic dysfunctions
- Quadratus lumborum muscle subcostal nerve—L1–L4 somatic dysfunctions

OTHER SOMATIC DYSFUNCTIONS

- Innominate dysfunction
- Pubic shear dysfunction
- Restriction and congestion of the ischial rectal fossa
- Dependent edema, especially of the lower extremities
- Thoracic outlet syndrome
- Carpal tunnel syndrome
- Increased lumbar lordosis
- Increased thoracic kyphosis
- Diaphragm restrictions

TREATMENT

 ### 2-MINUTE TREATMENT

- Head—OA release **M99.00**
- Lumbar—soft tissue, MET, MFR, and/or HVLA **M99.03**
- Sacral inhibition **M99.04**

 ### 5-MINUTE TREATMENT

- Innominate dysfunction—MET **M99.05**
- Innominate—pubic shear dysfunction: MET **M99.05**
- Sacral dysfunction—MET **M99.04**

 ### EXTENDED TREATMENT

- Lower extremity—psoas muscle: CS **M99.06**
- Lower extremity—piriformis: CS, MET **M99.06**
- Innominate—ischial rectal fossa: MFR **M99.05**
- Cervical—soft tissue, MFR, FPR, and/or HVLA **M99.01**
- Thoracic outlet syndrome **M99.01**, **M99.02**, and/or **M99.08**
- Thoracic—soft tissue, MET, MFR, and/or HVLA **M99.02**
- Lower extremity—pedal pump **M99.06**
- Abdomen/other—diaphragm: doming technique **M99.09**
- Thoracic lymphatic duct treatment **M99.09**
- Lower extremities—mild, slow effleurage/pétrissage of lower extremities **M99.06**
- Sacral rocking **M99.04**
- Abdomen/other/viscerosomatic—Chapman's reflexes for ovaries and uterus **M99.09**

P

Continued

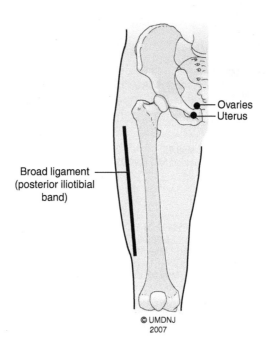

Ovaries
Uterus

Broad ligament
(posterior iliotibial
band)

© UMDNJ
2007

PREMENSTRUAL SYNDROME

 BASICS

DESCRIPTION

The physical and psychological symptoms some women experience in the week before menstruation. Symptoms may include bloating, headache, irritability, anxiety or depression, difficulty sleeping, fatigue, and breast swelling and tenderness.

 PHYSIOLOGY AND ASSOCIATED SOMATIC DYSFUNCTIONS

PARASYMPATHETICS

- Increased tone = vasodilation, nausea, vomiting, diarrhea
- Vagus nerve
  - ➤ Somatic dysfunctions of occipitoatlantal joint (OA), atlantoaxial joint (AA), C2
  - ➤ Compression of occipitomastoid sutures as well as OA joint
- Pelvic splanchnic nerves

SYMPATHETICS

- Increased tone = vasoconstriction, constipation, increased sensitivity to acid
- Somatic dysfunctions of T1–T4 and/or T5–L2
- Celiac ganglion—fascial restriction
- Superior mesenteric ganglion—fascial restriction
- Inferior mesenteric ganglion—fascial restriction

MOTOR

- Somatic dysfunctions of C2–C8 (levator scapulae muscle, scalene muscle)

 OTHER SOMATIC DYSFUNCTIONS

- Fascial restriction of ischial rectal fossa and sacral ligaments
- Innominate dysfunction

TREATMENT

 2-MINUTE TREATMENT

- Head—OA release **M99.00**
- Sacral base inhibition **M99.04**

 5-MINUTE TREATMENT

- Innominate dysfunction—MET **M99.05**
- Sacral dysfunctions—MET **M99.04**
- Sacral rocking technique **M99.04**

 EXTENDED TREATMENT

- Upper extremity—cervical levator scapulae muscle and scalene muscles: CS and/or MFR **M99.01** and/or **M99.07**
- Cervical—soft tissue, MFR, FPR, and/or HVLA **M99.01**
- Thoracic—soft tissue, MET, MFR, and/or HVLA **M99.02**
- Lumbar—soft tissue, MET, MFR, and/or HVLA **M99.03**
- Innominate—ischial rectal fossa: MFR **M99.05**
- Abdomen/other—ganglion restriction: MFR **M99.09**
- Abdomen/other/viscerosomatic—Chapman's reflexes for ovaries and uterus **M99.09**

P

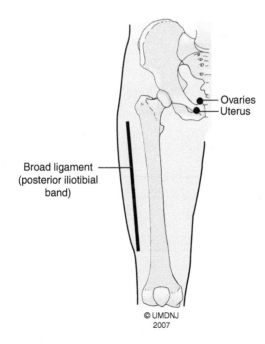

Ovaries
Uterus

Broad ligament
(posterior iliotibial
band)

© UMDNJ
2007

PYLORIC STENOSIS

BASICS

DESCRIPTION

Hypertrophy of the pyloric sphincter resulting in failure to thrive, GERD, and emesis

PHYSIOLOGY AND ASSOCIATED SOMATIC DYSFUNCTIONS

PARASYMPATHETICS

- Increased tone = increased acid production and peristalsis
- Vagus nerve (CN X) exits the jugular foramen (composed of occiput and temporal bones).
  ➤ Somatic dysfunctions of occipitoatlantal joint (OA), atlantoaxial joint (AA), C2
  ➤ Compression of occipitomastoid sutures

SYMPATHETICS

- Increased tone = decreased acid production and peristalsis
- Somatic dysfunction of T5–T10
- Prevertebral ganglion—fascial restriction
  ➤ Celiac ganglion

OTHER SOMATIC DYSFUNCTIONS

- Pyloric sphincter hypertonicity
- Diaphragm restriction of motion and at all attachments
- Cisterna chyli—fascial restriction
- Left thoracic duct fascial restriction

TREATMENT

 2-MINUTE TREATMENT

- Abdomen/other—celiac ganglion: MFR **M99.09**

 5-MINUTE TREATMENT

- Abdomen/other—pyloric sphincter: MFR **M99.09**
- Abdomen/other—mesenteric release **M99.09**

 EXTENDED TREATMENT

- Head—vagus nerve: OA release, V spread of occipitomastoid suture **M99.00**
- Cervical—MFR, FPR, and/or HVLA **M99.01**
- Thoracic—MFR, MET, and/or HVLA **M99.02**
- Abdomen/other—left thoracic duct: lymphatic **M99.09**
- Abdomen/other—diaphragm
  - ➤ Doming technique **M99.09**
  - ➤ Thoracolumbar junction—MET, MFR, HVLA **M99.02**, **M99.03**
- Abdomen/other—cisterna chyli: MFR (lymph) **M99.09**

P

RESTLESS LEGS SYNDROME

 BASICS

DESCRIPTION

Crampy, achy, gnawing, or burning, often painful, sensations in one or both lower extremities leading to a need to continually reposition the lower extremities to seek comfort

 PHYSIOLOGY AND ASSOCIATED SOMATIC DYSFUNCTIONS

PARASYMPATHETICS

Not applicable

SYMPATHETICS

- Increased tone = dilated arterioles of the muscles (cholinergic and adrenergic β2), constricted arterioles of the muscles (adrenergic α)
- Somatic dysfunction of T10–L2

MOTOR

- Gluteus maximus muscle L5–S2 irritating sciatic nerve
- Psoas muscle T12–L4 irritating iliohypogastric nerve, ilioinguinal nerve, genitofemoral nerve, lateral femoral cutaneous nerve, or femoral nerve
- Piriformis S1–S2 irritating sciatic nerve

 OTHER SOMATIC DYSFUNCTIONS

- Innominate tension on iliolumbar ligaments irritating superficial nerves of groin and lateral thigh
- Lumbar L4–L5 tight Iliolumbar ligaments
- Posterior fibular head irritating common peroneal nerve
- Hypertonicity of muscles of the lower extremity
- Ankle/foot dysfunctions

TREATMENT

 2-MINUTE TREATMENT

- Lower extremity—psoas muscle: MET, CS **M99.06**
- Lower extremity—piriformis muscle: MET, CS **M99.06**
- Lower extremity—muscles of the lower extremity: MFR **M99.06**

 5-MINUTE TREATMENT

- Lower extremity—posterior fibular head: BLT, MET, HVLA **M99.06**
- Lumbar—MET and/or HVLA **M99.03**

 EXTENDED TREATMENT

- Innominate dysfunction—MET **M99.05**
- Lower extremity—ankle/foot dysfunctions: MET and/or HVLA **M99.06**

R

RHINITIS, ALLERGIC

 BASICS

DESCRIPTION

Inflammation of the nasal mucosa with watery nasal secretions; may be associated with allergies, infection, medication use, and other environmental irritants

 PHYSIOLOGY AND ASSOCIATED SOMATIC DYSFUNCTIONS

PARASYMPATHETICS

- Increased tone = significantly increased secretions of nasal, lacrimal, and submandibular glands
- Facial nerve (CN VII), glossopharyngeal nerve (CN IX)—cranial dysfunction
- Vagus nerve
  ➤ Somatic dysfunctions of occipitoatlantal joint (OA), atlantoaxial joint (AA), C2
  ➤ Compression of occipitomastoid sutures as well as OA joint

SYMPATHETICS

- Increased tone = vasoconstriction and slight secretions of nasal, lacrimal, and submandibular glands
- Somatic dysfunctions of T1–T5

MOTOR

- Somatic dysfunctions of C3–C5 (phrenic nerve to the diaphragm; irritation caused by lung proximity)

 OTHER SOMATIC DYSFUNCTIONS

- Eustachian tube dysfunction
- Medial pterygoid muscle trigger point
- Masseter muscle trigger point
- Cranial dysfunction
- Lymphatic congestion of lymph nodes: preauricular and postauricular, submaxillary and submental, supraclavicular

TREATMENT

 2-MINUTE TREATMENT

- Head—supraorbital and infraorbital non-noxious massage **M99.00**
- Head—nasion gapping **M99.00**
- Head—frontal lift **M99.00**

 5-MINUTE TREATMENT

- Head—periauricular drainage technique **M99.00**
- Head—Muncie technique **M99.00**
- Abdomen/other/viscerosomatic—Chapman's reflex for ear and/or sinuses **M99.09**

 EXTENDED TREATMENT

- Head—decreased CRI: CV4 hold **M99.00**
- Head—vagus nerve: OA release **M99.00**
- Head—sphenopalatine ganglion stimulation **M99.00**
- Cervical—soft tissue, MFR, FPR, and/or HVLA **M99.01**
- Thoracic—soft tissue, MET, MFR, and/or HVLA **M99.02**

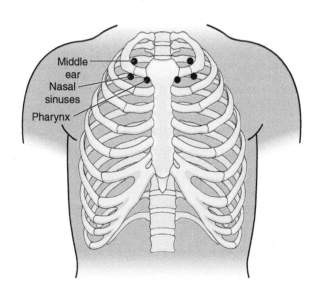

R

SACROILIITIS

 BASICS

DESCRIPTION

Inflammation of one or both sacroiliac joints that is caused by trauma, degenerative joint disease, or systemic inflammatory diseases such as ankylosing spondylitis; may cause pain in gluteal region, low back, and/or down one or both legs

 PHYSIOLOGY AND ASSOCIATED SOMATIC DYSFUNCTIONS

PARASYMPATHETICS

Currently under study
- Stimulation of peripheral, afferent vagus nerve fibers by endotoxin or cytokines can activate the hypothalamic–pituitary–adrenal (HPA) axis and sympathetic nervous system (SNS) centrally, resulting in peripheral release of anti-inflammatory glucocorticoids and norepinephrine (NE).
- May inhibit tumor necrosis factor (TNF)-α production by splenic macrophages via a signal from the celiac-superior mesenteric plexus projecting in the splenic nerve, which is composed principally of catecholaminergic fibers

SYMPATHETICS

- Regulatory function of the SNS includes monitoring and influencing immune homeostasis.
- Increased tone
  - ➤ Dilated arterioles of the muscles (cholinergic and adrenergic $\beta2$), constricted arterioles of the muscles (adrenergic α)
  - ➤ Stimulates catecholamine production in the different lymphoid organs via the efferent fibers, inhibits the development of a T helper (Th) 1 immune response, and shift the Th1/Th2 balance toward a Th2 immune response which is "humoral immunity" upregulation of antibody production to fight extracellular organisms
- Somatic dysfunction of T10–L2

MOTOR

- Piriformis hypertonicity and tenderness S1–S2
- Gluteus maximus muscle hypertonicity and tenderness inferior gluteal nerve L5–S2

 OTHER SOMATIC DYSFUNCTIONS

- Innominate dysfunction affecting sacral motion and tension on iliolumbar ligaments
- Lumbar L1–L5 tight iliolumbar ligaments

SPECIALIZED TESTING

- FABERE (Patrick's) test
- Lumbosacral spring test
- Trendelenburg's sign/hip drop test
- ASIS compression test or standing/seated flexion tests

 TREATMENT

 2-MINUTE TREATMENT

- Sacrum—ART **M99.04**
- Lower extremity—piriformis muscle: MET, CS **M99.06**

 5-MINUTE TREATMENT

- Sacrum—MET **M99.04**
- Lumbar—MET and/or HVLA **M99.03**

 EXTENDED TREATMENT

- Sacrum—sacral rocking, BLT **M99.04**
- Innominate dysfunction—MET **M99.05**

S

SCIATICA

 BASICS

DESCRIPTION

Pain along the course of a sciatic nerve especially in the back of the thigh caused by compression or inflammation of the nerve

 PHYSIOLOGY AND ASSOCIATED SOMATIC DYSFUNCTIONS

PARASYMPATHETICS

Not applicable

SYMPATHETICS

- Increased tone = dilated arterioles of the muscles (cholinergic and adrenergic β2), constricted arterioles of the muscles (adrenergic α)
- Somatic dysfunction of T10–L2

MOTOR

- Piriformis hypertonicity and tenderness S1–S2
- Gluteus maximus muscle hypertonicity and tenderness inferior gluteal nerve L5–S2
- Hamstring muscle hypertonicity and tenderness L4–S3 tibial nerve (common peroneal for short head of biceps femoris muscle)

 OTHER SOMATIC DYSFUNCTIONS

- Innominate dysfunction affecting sacral motion and tension on iliolumbar ligaments
- Lumbar L4–L5 tight iliolumbar ligaments
- Posterior fibular head irritating common peroneal nerve
- Tibia on talus dysfunction

 SPECIALIZED TESTING

- FABERE (Patrick's) test
- Leg raising
- Lumbosacral spring test
- Hip drop test
- Standing/seated flexion tests
- Thomas's test
- Trendelenburg's test

TREATMENT

 2-MINUTE TREATMENT

- Lower extremity—piriformis muscle: MET, CS **M99.06**
- Lower extremity—hamstring muscle: MFR **M99.06**

 5-MINUTE TREATMENT

- Lower extremity—posterior fibular head: HVLA **M99.06**
- Lumbar—MET and/or HVLA **M99.03**

 EXTENDED TREATMENT

- Innominate dysfunction—MET **M99.05**
- Lumbar—**M99.03**
- Lower extremity—ankle/foot dysfunctions: MET and/or HVLA **M99.06**
- Rule out causes of radiculopathy; counsel patient on stretching and exercise.

S

SCOLIOSIS

 BASICS

DESCRIPTION

Pathologic or functional lateral curvature of the spine

 PHYSIOLOGY AND ASSOCIATED SOMATIC DYSFUNCTIONS

PARASYMPATHETICS

Not applicable

SYMPATHETICS

May be affected by lateral curves at the paravertebral chain ganglion or by relative changes in rib motion due to anatomic proximity to rib head. Spinal level varies based on presentation.

MOTOR

May be affected by lateral curves. Rotoscoliosis will mimic Fryette's type I somatic dysfunctions.

 OTHER SOMATIC DYSFUNCTIONS

- Pelvic side shifting
- Apparent or actual leg length inequalities
- Sacral declination may cause functional scoliosis (Fryette's type I compensatory somatic dysfunctions).
- Fryette's type II somatic dysfunctions may lead to compensatory rotoscoliosis (Fryette's type I somatic dysfunctions).

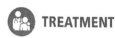 **TREATMENT**

Note: Look for anatomic leg length discrepancies if innominate and/or sacral findings do not make sense or if leg length appears short after treatment, particularly after several osteopathic manipulative medicine treatments. Consider also postural exercises as well as long restrictor muscle stretching prescription for symmetry to stretch muscles on side of concavity.

- Stretch hypertonic muscles
- Postural retraining then strengthening hypotonic musculature (Often, anterior musculature is hypertonic as well, particularly pectoralis muscles and iliopsoas.)
- Retraining and strengthening lower trapezius muscle and other muscles invested in thoracolumbar fascia

 2-MINUTE TREATMENT

- Innominate—MET **M99.05**
- Sacrum—MET **M99.04**

 5-MINUTE TREATMENT

- Thoracic—MET **M99.02**
- Lumbar—MET **M99.03**

 EXTENDED TREATMENT

- Thoracic—MFR and/or HVLA **M99.02**
- Lumbar—MFR and/or HVLA **M99.03**

S

SINUSITIS

 BASICS

DESCRIPTION

Infection (viral, bacterial, or fungal etiology) of the air sinuses of the head

 PHYSIOLOGY AND ASSOCIATED SOMATIC DYSFUNCTIONS

PARASYMPATHETICS

- Facial nerve (CN VII) via sphenopalatine ganglion
- Vagus nerve
  - ➤ Somatic dysfunctions of occipitoatlantal joint (OA), atlantoaxial joint (AA), C2
  - ➤ Compression of occipitomastoid sutures as well as OA joint

SYMPATHETICS

- Somatic dysfunctions of T1–T4

MOTOR

- Trigeminal nerve (CN V)—somatic afferents; somatosensory
- Tenderness/fascial restriction at supraorbital and infraorbital notch and over frontal and maxillary sinuses

 OTHER SOMATIC DYSFUNCTIONS

- Eustachian tube dysfunction
- Cranial dysfunction
- Lymphatic congestion of lymph nodes: preauricular and postauricular, submaxillary and submental, supraclavicular, and anterior cervical chain

TREATMENT

 2-MINUTE TREATMENT

- Head—supraorbital and infraorbital (CN V) massage **M99.00**
- Head—frontal and maxillary effleurage **M99.00**

 5-MINUTE TREATMENT

- Head—periauricular drainage technique **M99.00**
- Cervical—lymphatic drainage of anterior cervical lymphatics **M99.01**
- Abdomen/other/viscerosomatic—Chapman's reflexes: midmaxillary line above the clavicle for ear and below the clavicle for sinuses **M99.09**

 EXTENDED TREATMENT

- Head—OA: MFR **M99.00**
- Head—sphenopalatine ganglion stimulation **M99.00**
- Cervical—C2: soft tissue, MFR, FPR, and/or HVLA **M99.01**
- Thoracic—soft tissue, MET, MFR, and/or HVLA **M99.02**
- Rib raising **M99.08**
- Head—Muncie technique **M99.00**

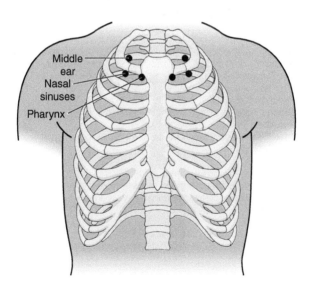

SPINAL STENOSIS

 BASICS

DESCRIPTION

Narrowing of central spinal canal or neural foramen resulting in impingement of the spinal cord or nerve roots that are adjacent. Symptoms include pain, numbness, tingling, and weakness depending on the severity. Osteopathic treatment is directed at improving function and reducing related somatic dysfunctions.

 ## PHYSIOLOGY AND ASSOCIATED SOMATIC DYSFUNCTIONS

Dysautonomia or imbalance of the autonomic nervous system may be associated with spinal stenosis related to the spinal segments involved in the disease process.

PARASYMPATHETICS

- Increased tone = reduced cardiac rate, respiratory system regulation, increased peristalsis, gallbladder wall contraction, contracted detrusor muscle of the bladder
- Vagus nerve
  - ➤ Somatic dysfunctions of occipitoatlantal joint (OA), atlantoaxial joint (AA), C2
  - ➤ Compression of occipitomastoid sutures as well as OA joint
- Pelvic splanchnic nerves S2–S4
  - ➤ Sacral torsions
  - ➤ Decreased sacral motion
  - ➤ Sacroiliac joint pain

SYMPATHETICS

- Increased tone = decreased kidney output, decreased peristalsis, gallbladder wall relaxation, relaxed detrusor muscle of the bladder, dilated arterioles of the muscles (cholinergic and adrenergic β2), constricted arterioles of the muscles (adrenergic α), pain (see Complex Regional Pain Syndrome [Reflex Sympathetic Dystrophy])
- Somatic dysfunctions of T1–L2
- Celiac ganglion—fascial restriction
- Superior mesenteric ganglion—fascial restriction
- Inferior mesenteric ganglion—fascial restriction

MOTOR

- Erector spinae muscle—segmental innervation C1–S5
- Gluteal muscles inferior and superior gluteal nerves
- Psoas muscle L1–L4 (Flexed posture may relieve nerve compression but may lead to somatic dysfunction and postural imbalance.)
- Piriformis S1–S2
- Quadratus lumborum muscle subcostal nerve L1–L4

SPECIALIZED TESTING

- Spurling test
- FABERE (Patrick's) test
- Straight leg raise test
- Lumbosacral spring test
- Hip drop test
- Standing/seated flexion tests
- Thomas's test
- Trendelenburg's test

 TREATMENT

 2-MINUTE TREATMENT

- Cervical—soft tissue and/or MET **M99.01**
- Lower extremity—psoas muscle: CS **M99.06**
- Lumbar spine—soft tissue, MFR, and/or MET **M99.03**

 5-MINUTE TREATMENT

- Cervical—FPR, CS, and/or MFR **M99.01**
- Innominate dysfunction—MET **M99.05**
- Sacral dysfunction—MET **M99.04**

 EXTENDED TREATMENT

- Lower extremity—piriformis: MET, CS **M99.06**
- Lower extremity—gluteal muscles: CS, MET **M99.06**
- Abdomen/other—diaphragm: doming technique **M99.09**
- Thoracic—soft tissue, MET, and/or MFR, **M99.02**
- Abdomen/other—ganglion restriction: MFR **M99.09**
- Abdomen/other/viscerosomatic—Chapman's reflexes for corresponding visceral dysfunctions **M99.09**

S

TACHYCARDIA

 BASICS

DESCRIPTION

An abnormally rapid beating of the heart, defined as a resting heart rate of 100 or more beats per minute in an average adult

 PHYSIOLOGY AND ASSOCIATED SOMATIC DYSFUNCTIONS

PARASYMPATHETICS

- Increased tone = bradycardia
- Vagus nerve (CN X) exits the jugular foramen (composed of occiput and temporal bones).
  - ➤ Somatic dysfunctions of occipitoatlantal joint (OA), atlantoaxial joint (AA), C2
  - ➤ Compression of occipitomastoid sutures

SYMPATHETICS

- Increased tone = tachycardia
- Somatic dysfunctions of T1–T5

MOTOR

- Somatic dysfunctions C3–C5 (phrenic nerve to the diaphragm; irritation caused by proximity to the heart)

 OTHER SOMATIC DYSFUNCTIONS

- Rib dysfunction
- Flattened diaphragm
- Scalene muscle hypertonicity and tenderpoints
- Pectoralis major muscle trigger point
- Pectoralis minor muscle hypertonicity and tenderpoints

TREATMENT

 ## 2-MINUTE TREATMENT

- Cervical—carotid massage (if hemodynamically stable) **M99.01**

 ## 5-MINUTE TREATMENT

- Upper extremity—right-sided pectoralis major muscle tenderpoint (clavicular head): CS **M99.07**
- Thoracic—HVLA **M99.02**

 ## EXTENDED TREATMENT

- Head—vagus nerve: OA release and/or V spread **M99.00**
- Cervical—scalene muscle: CS and/or MET **M99.01**
- Cervical—MFR, MET, and/or FPR **M99.01**
- Thoracic—MFR, DIR paravertebral muscles **M99.02**
- Rib dysfunction—MET **M99.08**
- Upper extremity—pectoralis minor muscles: CS and/or MFR **M99.07**
- Abdomen/other/viscerosomatic—diaphragm
  - ➤ Doming technique **M99.09**
  - ➤ Thoracolumbar junction: FPR, MET, MFR, HVLA **M99.02**, **M99.03**
- Abdomen/other/viscerosomatic—Chapman's reflex for heart **M99.09**

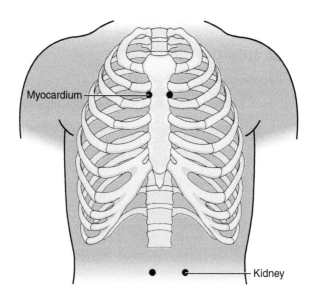

TEMPOROMANDIBULAR JOINT DYSFUNCTION

 BASICS

DESCRIPTION

A collection of symptoms caused either by dysfunction of the TMJ or spasm of the masticatory muscles that is often characterized by a clicking or popping sound of the jaw when moved and may include pain in the TMJ, facial pain, headache, earache, or neck pain

 PHYSIOLOGY AND ASSOCIATED SOMATIC DYSFUNCTIONS

PARASYMPATHETICS

- Increased tone = vasodilatation and copious secretions of submandibular glands
- Facial nerve (CN VII)
- Glossopharyngeal nerve (CN IX)
  ➤ Cranial strains
  ➤ Compression of occipitomastoid sutures as well as OA joint

SYMPATHETICS

- Increased tone = vasoconstriction and slight secretions of submandibular glands
- Somatic dysfunctions of T1–T5

MOTOR

- Genioglossal—hypoglossal nerve (CN XII); geniohyoid C1 via hypoglossal nerve (CN XII); mylohyoid, digastric muscle, medial pterygoid muscles: mandibular trigeminal nerve (CN V3)
  ➤ Tenderpoints
  ➤ Hypertonicity and restricted range of motion

 OTHER SOMATIC DYSFUNCTIONS

- Eustachian tube dysfunction
- Cranial dysfunction, especially temporal bone asymmetry
- Lymphatic congestion of lymph nodes: preauricular and postauricular, submaxillary and submental, supraclavicular
- Anterior fascial restriction of the cervical region down into sternum with resulting tenderpoints

TREATMENT

 2-MINUTE TREATMENT

- Head—direct inhibition of medial pterygoid, genioglossal, and digastric muscles **M99.00**

 5-MINUTE TREATMENT

- Head—mandibular MET technique **M99.00**
- Head—mental non-noxious massage **M99.00**
- Cervical—soft tissue, MFR, FPR, and/or HVLA **M99.01**

 EXTENDED TREATMENT

- Head—any cranial dysfunction **M99.00**
- Head—Muncie technique **M99.00**
- Head—periauricular drainage technique **M99.00**
- Head—OA release **M99.00**
- Cervical—anterior cervical: MFR **M99.01**
- Abdomen/other—sternum: CS, MFR **M99.09**
- Thoracic—soft tissue, MET, MFR, and/or HVLA **M99.02**
- Abdomen/other/viscerosomatic—Chapman's reflex for ear and/or sinuses **M99.09**

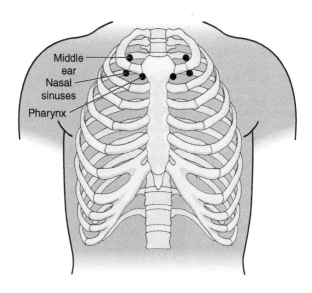

THORACIC OUTLET SYNDROME

 BASICS

DESCRIPTION

Pain or paresthesias of the upper extremity caused by compression or irritation of the brachial plexus or vascular structures of the thoracic outlet, which is outlined by the anterior and middle scalene muscles, the clavicle, the first rib, and possibly beneath the pectoralis minor muscle

 PHYSIOLOGY AND ASSOCIATED SOMATIC DYSFUNCTIONS

PARASYMPATHETICS

Not applicable

SYMPATHETICS

- Increased tone = dilated arterioles of the muscles (cholinergic and adrenergic β2), constricted arterioles of the muscles (adrenergic α)
- Somatic dysfunction of T5–T7

MOTOR

- Somatic dysfunction of C5–T1

 OTHER SOMATIC DYSFUNCTIONS

- Anterior and middle scalene muscle hypertonicity, tenderpoints, and restricted motion
- Somatic dysfunction of T1–T2
- Inhalation dysfunction of ribs 1 and 2
- Clavicle dysfunction
- Muscles of the upper extremity hypertonicity, tenderpoints, and restricted motion
  - ➤ Pectoralis major muscle
  - ➤ Pectoralis minor muscle
  - ➤ Levator scapulae muscle
  - ➤ Teres major muscle
  - ➤ Teres minor muscle
  - ➤ Latissimus dorsi muscle

TREATMENT

 2-MINUTE TREATMENT

- Thoracic—HVLA, MET **M99.02**

 5-MINUTE TREATMENT

- Ribs 1 and 2—FPR, MET, and/or HVLA **M99.08**
- Upper extremity—pectoralis minor muscle: CS, MET **M99.07**

 EXTENDED TREATMENT

- Cervical—anterior and middle scalene muscles: MET, CS, and/or MFR **M99.01**
- Cervical—FPR, MFR, and/or HVLA **M99.01**
- Thoracic—FPR **M99.02**
- Upper extremity—muscles with hypertonicity and tenderpoints: CS, MET **M99.07**
- Upper extremity—clavicle: BLT, MET **M99.07**

T

TINNITUS

 BASICS

DESCRIPTION
Perceived sound described as ringing, hissing, or roaring

 PHYSIOLOGY AND ASSOCIATED SOMATIC DYSFUNCTIONS

PARASYMPATHETICS
Not applicable

SYMPATHETICS
Not applicable

MOTOR
- Spinal accessory nerve (CN XI) to sternocleidomastoid muscle
- Mandibular trigeminal nerve (CN V3) to temporalis muscle
  ➤ Temporal bone cranial dysfunction

 OTHER SOMATIC DYSFUNCTIONS

- TMJ dysfunction
- Eustachian tube dysfunction
- Medial pterygoid muscle
- Masseter muscle
- Sternocleidomastoid muscle
- Cranial dysfunction, especially torsions and sidebending of the cranium
- Lymphatic congestion of lymph nodes—preauricular and postauricular, submaxillary and submental, supraclavicular

TREATMENT

 2-MINUTE TREATMENT

- Head—Muncie technique **M99.00**
- Head—periauricular drainage technique **M99.00**

 5-MINUTE TREATMENT

- Head—sphenopalatine ganglion stimulation **M99.00**
- Head—assess for and treat cranial strains **M99.00**

 EXTENDED TREATMENT

- Head—vagus nerve: OA release **M99.00**
- Head—assess and treat the CRI: CV4 hold **M99.00**
- Cervical—MFR, FPR, and/or HVLA **M99.01**
- Head—posterior digastric muscle: CS and/or direct inhibition **M99.00**
- Abdomen/other/viscerosomatic—Chapman's reflex for ear **M99.09**

T

TORTICOLLIS

 BASICS

DESCRIPTION

Stiff neck caused by spasmodic contraction of the neck muscles drawing the head to one side with the chin pointing to the other side. The muscles affected are principally those supplied by the spinal accessory nerve (CN XI).

 PHYSIOLOGY AND ASSOCIATED SOMATIC DYSFUNCTIONS

PARASYMPATHETICS

- Increased tone = vasodilation and copious secretions of submandibular glands
- Facial nerve (CN VII), glossopharyngeal nerve (CN IX)
  - ➤ Cranial strains
  - ➤ Compression of occipitomastoid sutures as well as OA joint

SYMPATHETICS

- Increased tone = vasoconstriction and slight secretions of submandibular glands
- Somatic dysfunctions of T1–T5

MOTOR

- Sternocleidomastoid muscle—spinal accessory nerve (CN XI) passes through the jugular foramen and the foramen magnum

 OTHER SOMATIC DYSFUNCTIONS

- Cranial dysfunction particularly at occipitomastoid suture and occipital compression
- Lymphatic congestion of lymph nodes: preauricular and postauricular, submaxillary and submental, supraclavicular
- Anterior fascial restriction of the cervical region down into sternum with resulting tenderpoints
- Trapezius muscle myospasm due to innervation by accessory nerve

TREATMENT

 2-MINUTE TREATMENT

- Cervical—soft tissue with attention to sternocleidomastoid muscle **M99.01**

 5-MINUTE TREATMENT

- Head—V spread technique at the occipitomastoid suture on side of restriction **M99.00**
- Head—OA release **M99.00**

 EXTENDED TREATMENT

- Head—OA: MET **M99.00**
- Cervical—soft tissue, MFR, FPR, MET, and/or HVLA **M99.01**
- Cervical—anterior cervical: MFR **M99.01**
- Thoracic (T1–T5)—soft tissue, MFR, MET, and/or HVLA **M99.02**
- Upper extremity—clavicle: CS, FPR, MFR **M99.07**

T

URINARY TRACT INFECTION

 BASICS

DESCRIPTION

An infection anywhere from the kidneys to the ureters, to the bladder, and to the urethra

 PHYSIOLOGY AND ASSOCIATED SOMATIC DYSFUNCTIONS

PARASYMPATHETICS

- Increased tone = normal ureteral peristalsis, bladder contraction (detrusor), bladder sphincter (trigone) relaxation
- Vagus nerve
  - ➤ Somatic dysfunctions of occipitoatlantal joint (OA), atlantoaxial joint (AA), C2
  - ➤ Compression of occipitomastoid sutures as well as OA joint
- Pelvic splanchnic nerves
- S2–S4 somatic dysfunctions
  - ➤ Sacral torsions
  - ➤ Decreased sacral motion
  - ➤ Sacroiliac joint pain

SYMPATHETICS

- Increased tone = ureter spasm, bladder (detrusor) relaxation, bladder sphincter (trigone) contraction
- Somatic dysfunctions of T10–L2
- Superior mesenteric ganglion—fascial restriction
- Inferior mesenteric ganglion—fascial restriction

 OTHER SOMATIC DYSFUNCTIONS

- Fascial restriction of ischial rectal fossa and sacral ligaments
- Restriction of ischial rectal fossa and sacral ligaments
- Restriction and tenderpoints of levator ani (puborectalis, pubococcygeus, and iliococcygeus)
- Innominate dysfunction
- Restriction and tenderpoints of psoas muscle
- Restriction and tenderpoints of piriformis

TREATMENT

 2-MINUTE TREATMENT

- Sacral base inhibition **M99.04**
- Head—OA release **M99.00**

 5-MINUTE TREATMENT

- Lower extremity—psoas muscle: CS **M99.06**
- Innominate dysfunction—MET **M99.05**

 EXTENDED TREATMENT

- Lower extremity—piriformis: CS, MET **M99.06**
- Innominate—ischial rectal fossa: MFR **M99.05**
- Cervical—soft tissue, MFR, FPR, and/or HVLA **M99.01**
- Thoracic—soft tissue, MET, MFR, and/or HVLA **M99.02**
- Lumbar—soft tissue, MET, MFR, and/or HVLA **M99.03**
- Lower extremity—pedal pump **M99.06**
- Abdomen/other—ganglion restriction: MFR **M99.09**
- Sacral torsion—MET **M99.04**
- Sacral rocking technique **M99.04**
- Abdomen/other/viscerosomatic—Chapman's reflexes for kidneys, ureters, and bladder **M99.09**

VERTIGO/LABYRINTHITIS

 BASICS

DESCRIPTION

Inflammation of the vestibular labyrinth often leading to vertigo, dizziness, and tinnitus

 PHYSIOLOGY AND ASSOCIATED SOMATIC DYSFUNCTIONS

PARASYMPATHETICS

Not applicable

SYMPATHETICS

- Somatic dysfunctions of T1–T4

MOTOR

- Spinal accessory nerve (CN XI) to sternocleidomastoid muscle
- Mandibular trigeminal nerve (CN V3) to temporalis muscle
  - ➤ Temporal bone cranial dysfunction

 OTHER SOMATIC DYSFUNCTIONS

- Eustachian tube dysfunction
- Medial pterygoid muscle
- Masseter muscle
- Clavicular portion of sternocleidomastoid muscle
- Cranial dysfunction, especially torsions and sidebending of the cranium
- Lymphatic congestion of lymph nodes—preauricular and postauricular, submaxillary and submental, supraclavicular

TREATMENT

 2-MINUTE TREATMENT

- Head—Muncie technique **M99.00**
- Head—periauricular drainage technique **M99.00**

 5-MINUTE TREATMENT

- Head—sphenopalatine ganglion stimulation **M99.00**
- Head—assess for and treat cranial strains **M99.00**

 EXTENDED TREATMENT

- Head—vagus nerve: OA release **M99.00**
- Head—assess and treat the CRI: CV4 hold **M99.00**
- Cervical—MFR, FPR, and/or HVLA **M99.01**
- Head—posterior digastric muscle: CS and/or direct inhibition **M99.00**
- Abdomen/other/viscerosomatic—Chapman's reflex for ear **M99.09**

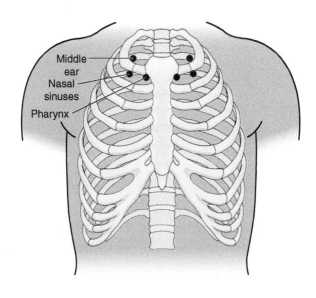

Section II

Structural Evaluations and Treatment Techniques

Diagnosing Somatic Dysfunction

GENERAL OVERVIEW OF SOMATIC DYSFUNCTION AND DIAGNOSIS

Somatic dysfunction is defined as "impaired or altered function of related components of the somatic (body framework) system: skeletal, arthrodial, and myofascial structures, and related vascular, lymphatic, and neural elements." The osteopathic mnemonic device for the most common findings in somatic dysfunction is TART:

Tenderness: unusual sensitivity to touch or pressure elicited from the patient by the osteopathic practitioner through palpation (the only subjective component)

Asymmetry: absence of symmetry of position or motion in corresponding parts opposite sides of the body that are normally alike; of particular use when describing position or motion alteration resulting from somatic dysfunction

Restricted motion: loss of range of motion

Tissue texture changes (TTC): a palpable change in tissues from skin to periarticular structures that represents any combination of the following signs: vasodilation, edema, flaccidity, hypertonicity, contracture, fibrosis as well as the following symptoms: itching, pain, tenderness, paresthesias. Types of TTCs include bogginess, thickening, stringiness, ropiness, firmness (hardening), increased/decreased temperature, and increased/decreased moisture.

Physiological motion of the spine: Fryette's laws

1. When the thoracic and lumbar spine are in a neutral position, the coupled motions of sidebending and rotation for a group of vertebrae are such that sidebending and rotation occur in opposite directions (with rotation occurring toward the convexity). Also known as type I somatic dysfunction and group dysfunctions because it often applies to a continuous series of dysfunctional vertebrae that are neutral (do not display a flexion or extension component to the somatic dysfunction).
2. When the thoracic and lumbar spine are sufficiently forward or backward bent (nonneutral), the coupled motions of sidebending and rotation in a single vertebral unit occur in the same direction. Also known as type II somatic dysfunction and single dysfunction because it often applies to a single dysfunctional vertebra that displays a flexion or extension component to the somatic dysfunction.
3. Initiating motion of a vertebral segment in any plane of motion will modify the movement of that segment in other planes of motion.

MOTIONS OF THE SPINE

CERVICAL SPINE

The **OA** joint is primarily responsible for flexion and extension. Its mechanics are such that it rotates in one direction and sidebends to the opposite side whether in neutral, flexion, or extension. If sidebending is restricted to the left, rotation will be restricted to the right and vice versa.

The **AA (C1–C2)** joint accounts for 50% of cervical rotation and is stabilized by the dens of C2.

Typical cervical vertebrae (C2–C7) follow type 2 Fryette's mechanics; that is, they rotate and sidebend toward the same side. C spine has no physiological neutral.

THORACIC AND LUMBAR SPINE

The thoracic and lumbar spine follow Fryette's laws as previously described.

INTERSEGMENTAL MOTION TESTING

CERVICAL SPINE

The **OA** joint
1. The patient lies supine on the treatment table.
2. Sit at the head of the table.
3. Place your index finger pads in front of the patient's ears, your thumbs at the top of the head, and your third digits under the base of the occiput.

Flexion/extension
4. Slowly flex and extend the patient's occiput in a rocking motion around an imaginary horizontal axis through the patient's ears without moving the rest of the cervical spine.

Sidebending and rotation
5. Translate the patient's occiput alternately to the left and right over C1 (atlas) without inducing any movement of C1–C7.
6. These steps are evaluated for asymmetric movement patterns that exhibit more sidebending in one direction and more rotation in the other and should be repeated in a flexed, neutral, and extended position. This is to determine which of these components is involved with the sidebending and rotational motions of the dysfunction.

The **AA (C1–C2)**
1. The patient lies supine with the head in neutral (if the patient's head is rotated, it will passively increase the rotational effect to that side).
2. Sit at the head of the table.
3. With the pads of the 2nd and 3rd index fingers, locate the articular pillars of C1 and C2
4. To localize to this joint, flex the entire neck to 45 degrees.
5. Rotate the head to the left. Stop rotation when C2 begins to rotate. This is the range of motion of C1 on C2 to the left.
6. Repeat the same motion for rotation right to assess the degrees of rotation.

Typical cervical vertebrae (C2–C7)
Rotation
1. The patient lies supine with the head in neutral (if the patient's head is rotated, it will passively increase the rotational effect to that side).
2. Sit at the head of the table and palpate articular pillars at each level with the pads of your index fingers alternating anterior springing pressure on the left and right articular pillars to evaluate for ease of left and right rotation rotational motion.
(If the right articular pillar moves anteriorly more easily and the left is resistant, the segment is rotating rotated left and the reverse is true.)

Sidebending
1. Typical cervicals follow type 2 Fryette's mechanics. Once the rotational component is determined, the sidebending is known; that is, they rotate and sidebend toward the same side.

Flexion/extension

1. The patient lies supine with the head in neutral (if the patient's head is rotated, it will passively increase the rotational effect to that side).
2. Sit at the head of the table and palpate articular pillars at each level with the pads of your index fingers.
3. With your index pads in place, note the prominence of rotation at the dysfunctional level.
4. Flex the patient's head forward and note whether the rotational component improves (becomes less prominent with ease of anterior pressure) or worsens (becomes more prominent with increased resistance to anterior pressure).
(If the rotational component improves in the flexed position, the dysfunction is termed flexed. If it worsens in this position, it is termed extended. Alternatively, the patient's head can be held off of the end of the table and extended to the level being evaluated. If the rotational component improves in the extended position, the dysfunction is termed extended. If it worsens in this position, it is termed flexed.)

THORACIC AND LUMBAR SPINE

Rotation

1. The patient is seated with the head in neutral (if the patient's head is rotated, it will passively increase the rotational effect to that side).
2. If the patient is seated, stand behind them and palpate the posterior component of the transverse processes at each level with the pads of your thumbs alternating anterior springing pressure on the left and right transverse processes to evaluate for ease of left and right rotation rotational motion.
(If the right transverse process moves anteriorly more easily and the left transverse process is resistant, the segment is rotating rotated left and the reverse is true.)

Sidebending

1. The patient is seated with the head in neutral (if the patient's head is rotated, it will passively increase the rotational effect to that side).
2. Stand behind them and palpate each level of the transverse processes with the pads of your thumbs on the posterolateral aspect of the transverse processes alternating a lateral force (translatory motion) left and right to evaluate for ease of left and right sidebending.
(If the thumb translates the segment more easily from left to right, the segment has its ease in left sidebending and is termed sidebent left and the reverse applies.)

Flexion/extension (applies to type II dysfunctions, i.e., single segment)

1. The patient is seated with the head in neutral (if the patient's head is rotated, it will passively increase the rotational effect to that side).
2. Stand behind them and palpate at the spinal level in question, with the pads of your thumbs on the posterior aspect of the transverse processes.
3. With your thumbs in place, note the prominence of rotation at the dysfunctional level.
4. Ask the patient to slowly bend forward and note whether the rotational component improves (becomes less prominent with ease of anterior pressure) or worsens (becomes more prominent with increased resistance to anterior pressure).
(If the rotational component improves in the flexed position, the dysfunction is termed flexed. If it worsens in this position, it is termed extended. Alternatively, the patient can arch their back at the level being evaluated. If the rotational component improves in the extended position, the dysfunction is termed extended. If it worsens in this position, it is termed flexed.)

Focused Structural Exams

INTRODUCTION

Focused structural exams are designed to be incorporated into the focused physical exam of the physician given a chief complaint from the patient. The areas listed to be assessed are not exhaustive but intended to give direction for high-yield areas of associated somatic dysfunction.

TART represents the four components for a somatic dysfunction:

Tissue texture changes

Asymmetry

Restriction of motion

Tenderness. Tenderness is the only subjective component and must be confirmed by the patient.

HEAD AND NECK COMPLAINTS (INCLUDE UPPER RESPIRATORY INFECTIONS, ALLERGIES, HEADACHE, NECK PAIN)

1. Head
   a. Evaluates cranial motion through vault hold
   b. Evaluates temporal mandibular joint motion
   c. Palpates frontal and maxillary sinuses for TART
   d. Evaluates passive motion of the OA
2. Cervical spine
   a. Evaluates active and passive range of motion (flexion/extension, rotation, sidebending)
   b. Palpates cervical spine for TART
3. Thoracic spine
   a. Evaluates active and passive range of motion (flexion/extension, rotation, sidebending)
   b. Palpates thoracic spine for TART
4. Upper extremity (shoulder)
   a. Evaluates passive motion of bilateral clavicles (flexion/extension, abduction/adduction, internal/ external rotation)
   b. Palpates and evaluates levator scapulae and trapezius muscle for TART
5. Ribs 1 to 4
   a. Evaluates active (through respiration) and passive range of motion
   b. Palpates ribs for TART

CARDIOPULMONARY SYMPTOMS

Although this focused structural exam has components in most regions of the body, emphasis should be given to body regions based on a patient's differential diagnosis.

1. Head: evaluates passive motion of the OA

2. Cervical: palpates cervical spine for TART

3. Thoracic spine: palpates thoracic spine for TART

4. Rib

    a. Evaluates active (through patient respirations) and passive range of motion of all ribs

    b. Palpates ribs, sternum, and associated muscles for TART including pectoralis major, pectoralis minor, serratus anterior, internal and external oblique muscles

5. Upper extremity

    a. Shoulder

        i. Evaluates passive motion of bilateral clavicles (flexion/extension, abduction/adduction, internal/external rotation)

6. Abdomen: evaluates respiratory diaphragm motion active (through patient respirations) and passive

7. Pelvis (related because of abdominal muscles attached to ribs)

    a. Performs ASIS compression or standing flexion tests

    b. Evaluates ASIS and PSIS positions (anterior/posterior rotations, inflares/outflares, shears)

8. Lower extremity: evaluates lower extremities for edema

Focused Structural Exams

GASTROINTESTINAL COMPLAINTS

1. Head: evaluates passive motion of the OA
2. Cervical: palpates cervical spine for TART
3. Thoracic spine
   a. Evaluates motion of thoracic outlet of patient
   b. Palpates thoracic spine for TART
4. Abdomen: evaluates respiratory diaphragm motion active (through patient respirations) and passive
5. Pelvis (related because of abdominal muscles attached to ribs)
   a. Performs ASIS compression or standing flexion tests
   b. Evaluates ASIS and PSIS positions (anterior/posterior rotations, inflares/outflares, shears)
6. Sacrum
   a. Performs seated flexion test
   b. Palpates sacral bases and inferior lateral angles (ILAs)
7. Lower extremity
   a. Palpates iliotibial band for TART
   b. Piriformis
      i. Evaluates motion with FAIR test
      ii. Evaluates for tenderness

LOW BACK PAIN
(INCLUDING PREGNANCY MODIFICATION)

1. Thoracic spine
   a. Evaluates active and passive range of motion (flexion/extension, rotation, sidebending)
   b. Palpates thoracic spine for TART
2. Lumbar spine
   a. Evaluates active and passive range of motion (flexion/extension, rotation, sidebending)
   b. Palpates lumbar spine for TART
3. Pelvis
   a. Evaluates active and passive motion of hips (flexion/extension, abduction/adduction, internal/external rotation)
   b. Performs ASIS compression or standing flexion tests
   c. Evaluates ASIS and PSIS positions (anterior/posterior rotations, inflares/outflares, shears)
   d. Externally palpates pelvic floor for restriction and tenderness
4. Sacrum
   a. Performs seated flexion test
   b. Palpates sacral bases and ILAs
      Pregnancy modifications
   c. Performs seated flexion test with knees apart to accommodate gravid abdomen
   d. Evaluates sacral bases and ILAs in lateral recumbent position
5. Lower extremity
   a. Muscle evaluation
      i. Psoas: evaluates psoas range of motion with Thomas's test and evaluates for tenderness
      ii. Piriformis: evaluates range of motion with FAIR test and evaluates for tenderness
      iii. Adductors: evaluates range of motion with FABER test and evaluates for tenderness
      iv. Hamstring: evaluates range of motion with straight leg raising and evaluates for tenderness
   b. Evaluates leg length by comparing medial malleoli positions
6. Gait evaluation: assesses for stance, stride and fluidity, and stability

Focused Structural Exams

LOWER EXTREMITY PAIN
(INCLUDES HIP, KNEE, ANKLE, FOOT)

1. Pelvis
   a. Evaluates active and passive motion of hips (flexion/extension, abduction/adduction, internal/external rotation)
   b. Performs ASIS compression or standing flexion tests
   c. Evaluates ASIS and PSIS positions
2. Lower extremity
   a. Muscle evaluation
      i. Psoas: evaluates psoas range of motion with Thomas's test and evaluates for tenderness
      ii. Piriformis: evaluates range of motion with FAIR test and evaluates for tenderness
      iii. Adductors: evaluates range of motion with FABER test and evaluates for tenderness
      iv. Hamstring: evaluates range of motion with straight leg raising and evaluates for tenderness
   b. Evaluates range of motion and tenderness of fibular head (affecting knee and ankle)
   c. Evaluates range of motion and tenderness of foot
      i. Mortise joint (dorsiflexion/plantarflexion)
      ii. Subtalar joint (inversion/eversion)
      iii. Midfoot (pronation/supination)
      iv. Forefoot (flexion/extension)
3. Gait evaluation: assesses for stance, stride, and fluidity and stability

UPPER EXTREMITY PAIN
(INCLUDES SHOULDER, ELBOW, WRIST, AND HAND)

1. Cervical spine
   a. Evaluates active and passive range of motion (flexion/extension, rotation, sidebending)
   b. Palpates cervical spine for TART
2. Thoracic spine
   a. Evaluates active and passive range of motion (flexion/extension, rotation, sidebending)
   b. Palpates thoracic spine for TART
3. Upper extremity
   a. Shoulder
      i. Evaluates active and passive motion of shoulders (flexion/extension, abduction/adduction, internal/external rotation); may do seated or lateral recumbent as 7 Stages of Spencer
      ii. Evaluates passive motion of bilateral clavicles (flexion/extension, abduction/adduction, internal/external rotation)
      iii. Palpates and evaluates superficial bilateral shoulder muscles while asking for tenderness
         1. Biceps
         2. Deltoid
         3. Latissimus dorsi
         4. Pectoralis major/minor
         5. Serratus Anterior
         6. Supraspinatus
         7. Trapezius
         8. Triceps
   b. Elbow/forearm
      i. Evaluates range of motion (flexion/extension, supination/pronation)
      ii. Evaluates radial head motion
      iii. Palpates for TART of forearm flexors and extensors
   c. Wrist
      i. Evaluates range of motion (flexion/extension, abduction/adduction)
      ii. Palpates for TART including carpal bone positioning
   d. Hand: palpates for TART
4. Ribs 1 to 8
   a. Evaluates active and passive range of motion
   b. Palpates ribs for TART

Focused Structural Exams

Techniques

OA RELEASE

1. The patient lies supine.
2. While seated at the head of the table, place your 2nd to 4th finger pads caudad to the base of the occiput.
3. Apply a mild cephalward traction to separate the occiput at the condyles from the atlas (C1) until there is a softening of tension.

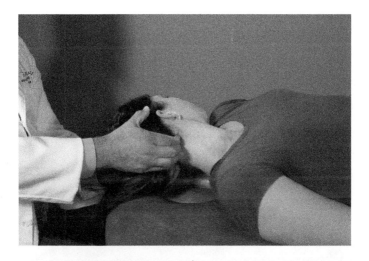

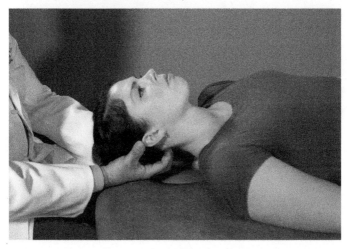

SINUS EFFLEURAGE

FRONTAL SINUS

1. The patient lies supine.

2. While seated at the head of the table, place your 2nd and 3rd finger pads just above the supraorbital ridges at the center of the frontal bone such that your 2nd digits are next to each other.

3. Following the shape of the frontal bones (lateral in direction), apply a slow (3 seconds per motion), gentle stroking pressure bilaterally stopping at the lateral aspect of the orbits.

4. Repeat this motion for 30 seconds to 2 minutes.

MAXILLARY SINUS

1. The patient lies supine.

2. While seated at the head of the table, place your 2nd and 3rd finger pads just inferior to the medial infraorbital ridge.

3. Following the shape of the maxillary bones (superior–medial to inferior–lateral in direction), apply a slow (3 seconds per motion), gentle stroking pressure bilaterally stopping just above the upper dentition.

4. Repeat this motion for 30 seconds to 2 minutes.

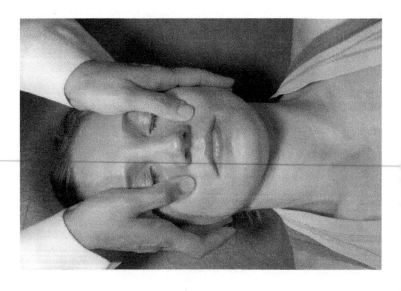

MUNCIE TECHNIQUE

1. The patient lies supine.
2. Stand at the side of the patient.
3. With the index finger of your gloved hand, palpate the palatine tonsillar region.
4. Apply a gentle lateral pressure with a rotatory motion (emphasis on inferior traction of the motion) for 15 to 20 seconds. Patients may exhibit a gag reflex. Short quick breathes by the patient while the technique is being performed should alleviate this.

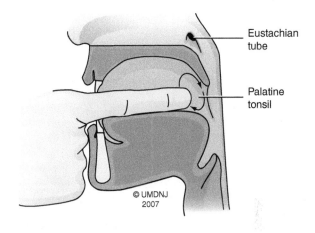

Eustachian tube

Palatine tonsil

© UMDNJ
2007

PTERYGOID RELEASE TECHNIQUE

1. The patient lies supine.
2. Stand at the side of the patient and place your cephalad hand on the forehead to stabilize the head.
3. Instruct the patient to open his or her mouth slowly.
4. With a gloved hand, place index finger of your caudad hand between the molars and the ramus of the mandible.
5. Apply a gentle posterior force (posterior–superior for lateral pterygoid and posterior–inferior for medial pterygoid).
6. Increase your pressure to match areas of hypertonicity in the pterygoid muscles (but only to patient tolerance).
7. Hold pressure for 10 to 20 seconds.

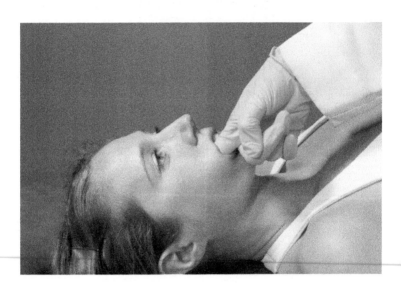

TMJ UNWINDING

1. The patient is seated.

2. Stand in front of the patient.

3. Ask the patient to open his or her mouth and relax the jaw.

4. With gloved hands, place thumbs on top of the patient's lower molars and grasp the outer mandible with rest of hands.

5. Apply a gentle anterior and inferior traction to disengage both TMJ joints for 10 to 30 seconds.

6. Allow the myofascial structures to unwind.

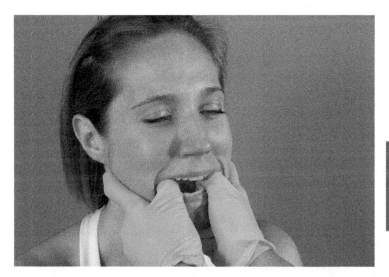

Techniques

GALBREATH TECHNIQUE

1. The patient lies supine.
2. Stand at the side of head of the patient, opposite to the side to be treated.
3. Place your cephalad hand on the forehead of the patient to stabilize the head.
4. Instruct the patient to open his or her mouth slightly to allow slack in the jaw.
5. Place 2nd and 3rd finger pads of your caudad hand on the posterior aspect of the angle of the mandible.
6. Apply anterior–medial traction of the mandible for approximately 3 to 5 seconds and then release.
7. Repeat Step 6 3–5 times.
8. Reassess.

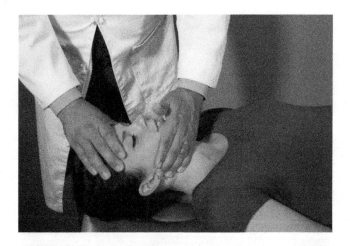

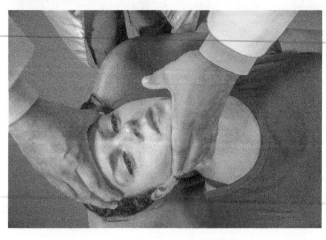

AURICULAR DRAINAGE

1. The patient lies supine.

2. Stand at the side of the patient's head, opposite the dysfunction.

3. Place your cephalad hand on the forehead of the patient to stabilize the head.

4. Separate your 2nd and 3rd fingers on your caudad hand and place the dysfunctional ear between the separated fingers.

5. Gently apply a clockwise motion to the dysfunctional ear for 10 to 20 seconds and then a counterclockwise motion with a force deep enough to engage the tissues also for 10 to 20 seconds.

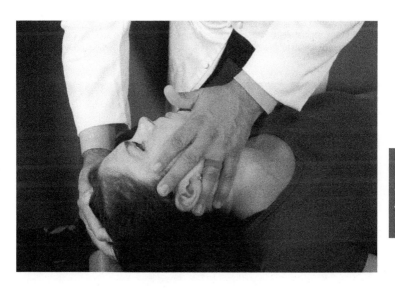

Techniques

VENOUS SINUS DRAINAGE

1. The patient lies supine.
2. Sit at the head of the table with your forearms resting on the table.
3. Palpate the patient's cranium over the area of the venous sinus to be treated.
4. Apply a gentle pressure along the path of the venous sinus, with particular focus on areas of increased tension until a release (softening) is felt.
   a. Transverse sinus drainage: Place your 2nd to 4th finger pads of both hands across the superior nuchal line.
   b. Confluence of sinuses: Support the patient's head at the occiput with one hand such that the 3rd finger pad rests on the inion (use your other hand if needed to stabilize the head).
   c. Occipital sinus: Place the 2nd to 4th finger pads of both hands along the midline of the occiput from the inion to the suboccipital tissues.
   d. Superior sagittal sinus: Place two crossed thumbs at lambda and exert opposing forces with each thumb to disengage the suture for 3 to 5 seconds, repeating toward bregma.

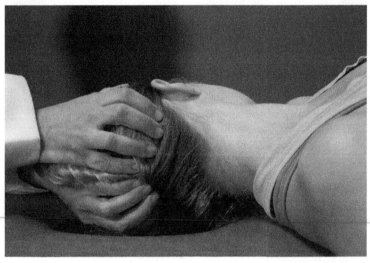

(continued)

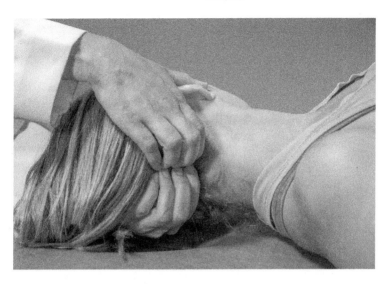

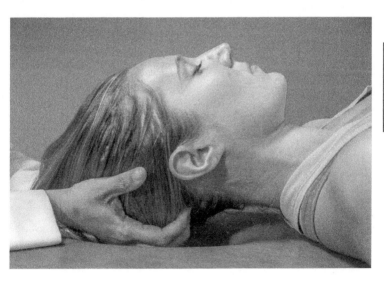

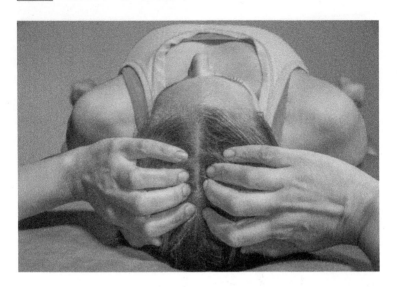

CV4 TECHNIQUE

1. The patient lies supine.
2. Sit at the head of the patient.
3. Create a cup with your hands such that your fingers overlap.
4. Cradle the skull in your hands with your thenar eminences against the occiput just medial to the occipitomastoid suture and your fingers near the base of the occiput.
5. Using the CRI, follow the occiput into the extension phases and resist the occiput motion during the flexion phases until a still point is reached.
6. Hold the occiput at the still point for several cycles.
7. Release from the still point and allow restoration of the normal flexion/extension movement in the occiput.

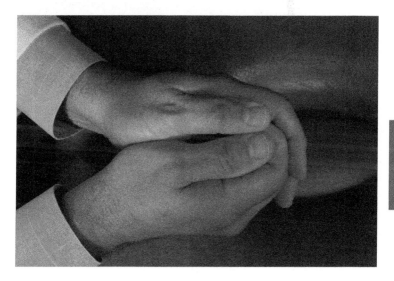

Techniques

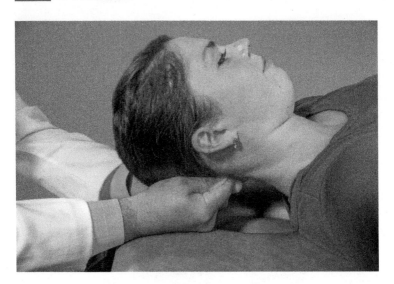

COUNTERSTRAIN—ANTERIOR TENDERPOINTS

1. The patient lies supine.
2. Sit at the head of the patient and identify the most tender anterior tenderpoint.
3. Locate the anterior tenderpoint with your index finger (the monitoring finger must remain unmoved for the duration of the treatment).
4. Direct the patient to assign the initial tenderness as 100% to however much tenderness is felt by the patient.
5. Use the opposite hand to cup the occiput and provide the necessary head support for positional changes.
6. Place the head and neck into flexion, with slight sidebending away and rotation away from the tenderpoint. *Maverick anterior tenderpoint AC7 treatment position is sidebending toward rotation away from tenderpoint.
7. Readjust the position to achieve the position of least tenderness with a goal of <30% of original tenderness.
8. Hold this position for 90 seconds or until a palpable release is achieved.
9. Passively return patient back to neutral position without the help of the patient.
10. Reassess for tenderness.

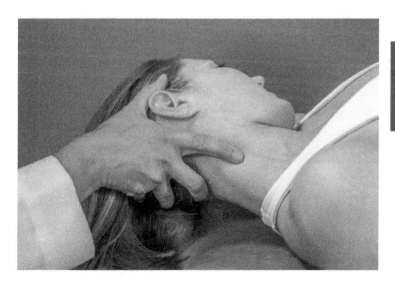

Techniques

FPR—ANTERIOR TENDERPOINTS

Steps 1–3 are the same as counterstrain

1. After the position of least tenderness is found, apply a facilitating vector force on top of the head through the axial skeleton in a direction through the cervical spine to the level of the tenderpoint.
2. Hold the position for 3 to 5 seconds while the soft tissue involving the tenderpoint releases.
3. Passively bring the patient back into a neutral position without the help of the patient and then release the facilitating force.
4. Reassess.

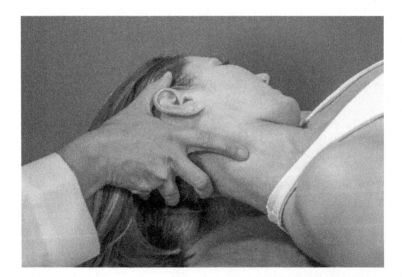

COUNTERSTRAIN—POSTERIOR TENDERPOINTS

1. The patient lies supine.

2. Sit at the head of the patient and identify the most tender posterior tenderpoint.

3. Locate the posterior tenderpoint with your index finger (the monitoring finger must remain unmoved for the duration of the treatment).

4. Direct the patient to assign the initial tenderness as 100% to however much tenderness is felt by the patient.

5. Use the opposite hand to cup the occiput and provide the necessary head support for positional changes. The patient's supported head may hang off the table to allow for further extension if needed.

6. Place the head and neck into extension, with slight sidebending away and rotation away from the tenderpoint. *Maverick posterior tenderpoint posterior C1 inion treatment position is flexion.

7. Readjust the position to achieve the position of least tenderness with a goal of <30% of original tenderness. Hold this position for 90 seconds or until a palpable release is achieved.

8. Passively return patient back to neutral position without the help of the patient.

9. Reassess.

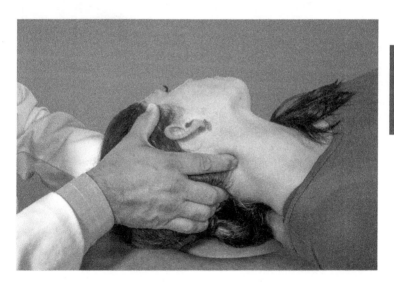

FPR—POSTERIOR TENDERPOINTS

Steps 1–3 are the same as counterstrain

1. After the position of least tenderness is found, apply a facilitating vector force on top of the head through the axial skeleton in a direction through the cervical spine to the level of the tenderpoint.

2. Hold the position for 3 to 5 seconds while the soft tissue involving the tenderpoint releases.

3. Passively bring the patient back into a neutral position without the help of the patient and then release the facilitating force.

4. Reassess.

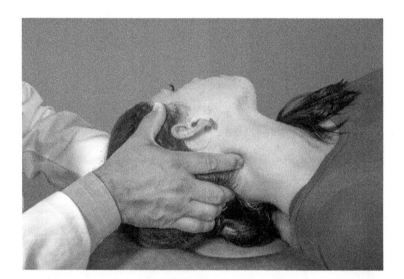

MUSCLE ENERGY—TYPICAL: C2–C7

1. The patient lies supine.
2. Stand at the head of the patient and place the second MCP of your hand on the side of the dysfunction on the articular pillar of the dysfunction.
3. Flex or extend to the level of the dysfunctional segment.
4. Rotate the head away from the side of rotational component of the dysfunction.
5. Induce sidebending away from the side of the rotational component of the dysfunction.
6. Further introduce rotation and sidebending, contacting the restrictive barrier while maintaining the necessary extension or flexion.
7. Instruct the patient to turn his or her head toward the direction of the dysfunction, against your isometric resistance, for 3 to 5 seconds.
8. Instruct the patient to rest.
9. After 1 second, take up any rotation and sidebending to contact the new restrictive barrier. Repeat the above steps, each time taking the patient's neck further into the direction of the restriction.
10. At the end of three to five cycles, take the patient into a final stretch toward the barrier.
11. Return to neutral and reevaluate for motion and symmetry of the segment.

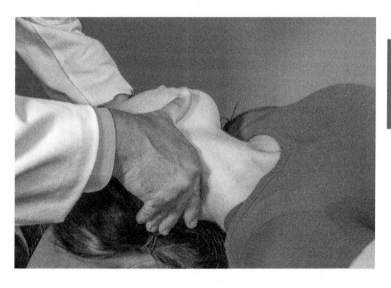

Techniques

MUSCLE ENERGY—ATYPICALS: AA

1. The patient lies supine.
2. Sit at the head of the patient and, upon identifying restriction at the AA, bring the cervical vertebrae back into a neutral position to avoid injury to the dens.
3. Place the second MCP of the hand on the side of the dysfunction on the patient's AA joint at the C1 transverse process while the thumb contacts the patient's mandible or zygomatic process.
4. Introduce rotation away from the side of the diagnosis, contacting the restrictive barrier.
5. Instruct the patient to turn his or her head toward the direction of the dysfunction, against your isometric resistance, for 3 to 5 seconds.
6. Instruct the patient to rest.
7. After 1 second, take up any rotation to contact the new restrictive barrier.
8. Repeat steps 3 to 6, each time taking the patient's neck further into the restrictive barrier.
9. At the end of three to five cycles, take the patient into a final stretch toward the barrier.
10. Return to neutral and reevaluate for motion of the segment.

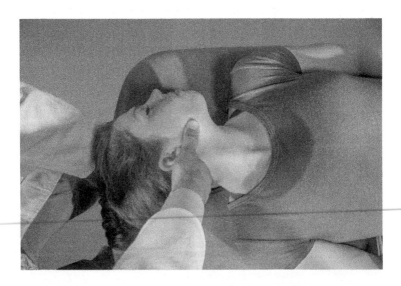

MUSCLE ENERGY—ATYPICALS: OA

1. The patient lies supine.
2. Stand at the head of the patient and place the second MCP of the hand on the posterior-lateral occipital bone on the side of the rotational component of the somatic dysfunction.
3. Sidebend the patient's OA away from the sidebending component of the dysfunction.
4. Rotate the head away from the rotational component of the dysfunction.
5. Flex or extend the head away from the flexion/extension component of the dysfunction.
6. Instruct the patient to move his or her head toward the direction of the dysfunction, against your isometric resistance for 3 to 5 seconds.
7. Instruct the patient to rest.
8. After 1 second, take up any motion in all three planes to contact the new restrictive barrier.
9. Repeat steps 3 to 6, each time taking the patient's head further into the direction of restriction.
10. At the end of three cycles, take the patient into a final stretch toward the barrier.
11. Return to neutral and reassess.

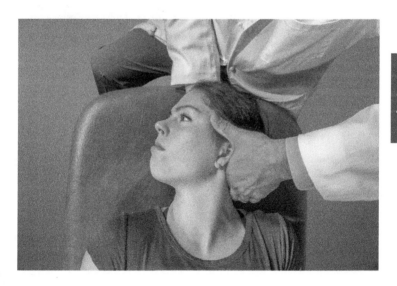

SOFT TISSUE—PERPENDICULAR STRETCH

1. The patient lies supine.
2. Sit or stand at the side of the patient at the level of the cervical spine.
3. Place your cephalad hand on the forehead to stabilize the patient's head and place the other hand on the opposite paravertebral musculature of the cervical spine.
4. Apply enough force to engage the deep myofascial structures.
5. Apply traction laterally and anteriorly (perpendicular to the spine) lasting approximately 3 seconds per cycle.

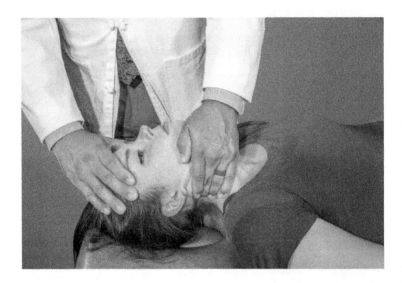

SOFT TISSUE—LONGITUDINAL STRETCH

1. The patient lies supine.
2. Sit or stand at the head of the patient.
3. Place hands on both sides of the posterior paravertebral musculature of the cervical spine. Apply sufficient force to engage the deep myofascial structures.
4. Apply traction longitudinally (along the length of the spine) lasting approximately 3 seconds per cycle.

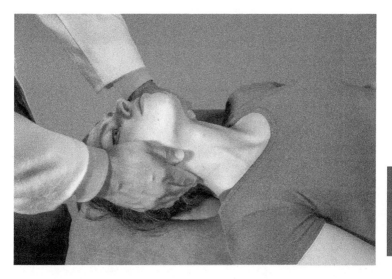

Techniques

HVLA—TYPICALS: C2–C7
(ROTATIONAL THRUST EMPHASIS)

1. The patient lies supine.
2. Stand at the head of the patient and place the second MCP of the hand on the side of the dysfunction on the articular pillar at the level of the somatic dysfunction.
3. Flex the head and neck to the level of the dysfunction.
4. Rotate the head away from the rotational component of the dysfunction.
5. Sidebend the head and neck toward the rotational component of the dysfunction.
6. Further introduce rotation and sidebending until you contact the restrictive barrier.
7. Give the rotational thrust through the articular pillar.
8. Return patient to neutral position.
9. Reassess.

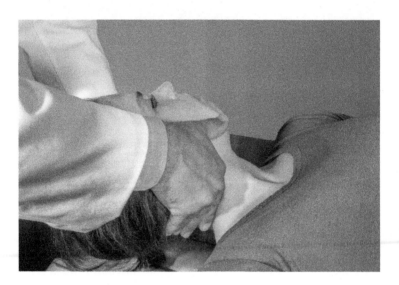

HVLA—ATYPICALS: AA

1. The patient lies supine.
2. To avoid injury to the dens, do not use any amount of flexion.
3. Sit at the head of the patient and place the second MCP on the side of dysfunction (thrusting hand) on the patient's AA joint contacting the C1 transverse process.
4. Introduce rotation, contacting the restrictive barrier.
5. Make a rotational thrust through the restrictive barrier.
6. Reassess.

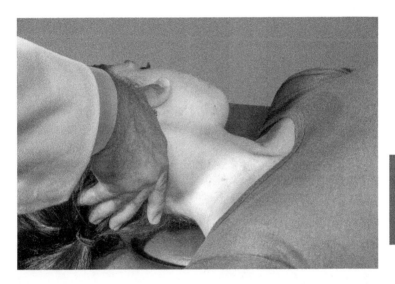

Techniques

HVLA—ATYPICALS: OA

1. The patient lies supine.
2. Stand at the head of the patient and place the second MCP on the OA joint on the side of the rotational component of the somatic dysfunction, contacting the occiput.
3. Sidebend the patient's OA toward the rotational component of the dysfunction.
4. Rotate the OA away from the rotational component of the dysfunction.
5. Flex or extend into the barrier by gliding on the OA condyles.
6. Thrust is rotational, toward the ipsilateral eye.
7. Return to neutral position.
8. Reassess.

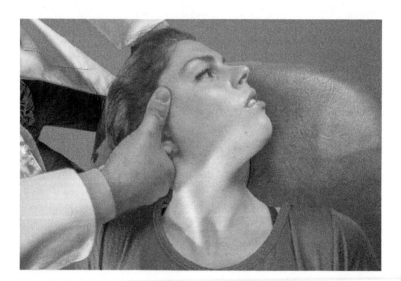

SEATED FORWARD LEANING ARTICULATORY

1. Stand in front of the patient slightly to one side. (If you have an adjustable table, lower it such that the top of his or her head is at the level of your chin.)
2. Have the patient lean forward, cross his or her arms at the wrists and rest his or her extended forearms on your shoulder that is closest to the midline.
3. Reach around his or her back and contact the transverse process with your finger pads.
4. Apply an anterior–superior springing force to the levels being treated for 20 to 40 seconds.

Techniques

COUNTERSTRAIN—ANTERIOR TENDERPOINTS

AT1–7

1. The patient lies supine.
2. Stand at the head of the patient.
3. Locate the tenderpoint with your index finger (the monitoring finger must remain unmoved for the duration of the treatment).
4. Direct the patient to assign the initial tenderness as 100% to however much tenderness is felt by the patient.
5. Flex the patient by lifting the head with your opposite hand or placing your flexed knee under the thoracic region until you find the position where the tenderpoint is least tender (at least 70% reduction according to the patient).
6. Shortening of surrounding muscles may help in the reduction of tenderness. This can be achieved by
   a. Sidebending of the cervical spine or thoracic spine
   b. Mobilization of the upper extremities: abduction/adduction, internal/external rotation
7. Readjust the position to achieve the position of least tenderness with a goal of <30% of original tenderness.
8. Hold this position for 90 seconds or until a palpable release is achieved.
9. Passively return to neutral.
10. Reassess tenderpoint.

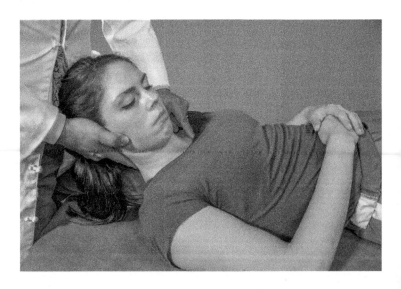

AT8–12

1. The patient lies supine.
2. Stand at the side of the patient.
3. Locate the tenderpoint with your index finger (the monitoring finger must remain unmoved for the duration of the treatment).
4. Direct the patient to assign the initial tenderness as 100% to however much tenderness is felt by the patient.
5. Flex the patient's hips and knees.
6. Place your caudad foot on the table and rest his or her lower legs on your thigh. Increase flexion of the patient's hips until you find the position where the tenderpoint is least tender (additional sidebending and rotation may assist in tenderness reduction). This can be achieved by rotating the patient's knees toward you (rotation of the spine) or bringing the ankles of the patient toward you (sidebending of the spine).
7. Readjust the position to achieve the position of least tenderness with a goal of <30% of original tenderness.
8. Hold this position for 90 seconds or until a palpable release is achieved.
9. Passively return to neutral.
10. Reassess tenderpoint.

COUNTERSTRAIN—POSTERIOR TENDERPOINTS

PT1–4

1. The patient lies supine with the head, neck, and upper back off the upper edge of the table.
2. Sit at the head of the table supporting the patient's head to prevent extension.
3. Locate the tenderpoint with your index finger (the monitoring finger must remain unmoved for the duration of the treatment).
4. Direct the patient to assign the initial tenderness as 100% to however much tenderness is felt by the patient.
5. Extend the patient's head, neck, and upper back to the level of the dysfunction. You may further reduce tenderness by sidebending and rotating away the head and neck.
6. Readjust the position to achieve the position of least tenderness with a goal of <30% of original tenderness.
7. Hold this position for 90 seconds or until a palpable release is achieved.
8. Passively return to neutral.
9. Reassess tenderpoint.

PT5–9

1. The patient lies prone.
2. Sit at the side of the tenderpoint.
3. Have the patient rotate his or her head/neck to the side opposite tenderpoint.
4. Locate the tenderpoint with your index finger (the monitoring finger must remain unmoved for the duration of the treatment).
5. Direct the patient to assign the initial tenderness as 100% to however much tenderness is felt by the patient.
6. Reach across the patient and lift his or her opposite shoulder, posterior and caudad. This causes extension, rotation away, and sidebending away from the side of the tenderpoint.
7. Readjust the position to achieve the position of least tenderness with a goal of <30% of original tenderness.
8. Hold this position for 90 seconds or until a palpable release is achieved.
9. Passively return to neutral.
10. Reassess tenderpoint.

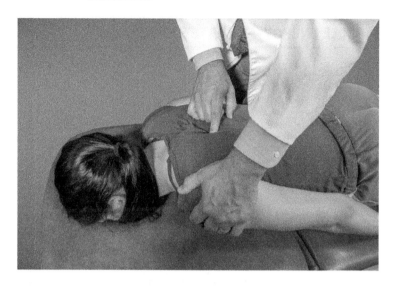

PT10–12

1. The patient lies prone.
2. Stand on the opposite side of the tenderpoint.
3. Locate the tenderpoint with your index finger (the monitoring finger must remain unmoved for the duration of the treatment).
4. Direct the patient to assign the initial tenderness as 100% to however much tenderness is felt by the patient.
5. Grasp the ASIS on the side of the tenderpoint and lift upward to induce extension and rotation of the pelvis.
6. Readjust the position to achieve the position of least tenderness with a goal of <30% of original tenderness.
7. Hold this position for 90 seconds or until a palpable release is achieved.
8. Passively return to neutral.
9. Reassess tenderpoint.

Techniques

MUSCLE ENERGY—FRYETTE'S TYPE 1

1. The patient is seated.
2. Stand behind the patient.
3. Have the patient grasp his or her elbows.
4. Place your thenar eminence over the rotated side of dysfunction.
5. With your other hand, reach under and then over the patient's folded arms and grasp the upper arm (on the side of the rotational dysfunction).
6. Sidebend and rotate (should be in opposite directions) the patient into the barrier.
7. Have the patient gently turn his or her body back against your resisting force.
8. The patient holds the contractive force for 3 to 5 seconds and then relaxes.
9. Pause for 1 to 2 seconds.
10. Repeat steps 6 to 8 a total of three to five times.
11. Take the patient into a final stretch toward the barrier and then return the patient to neutral.
12. Reassess.

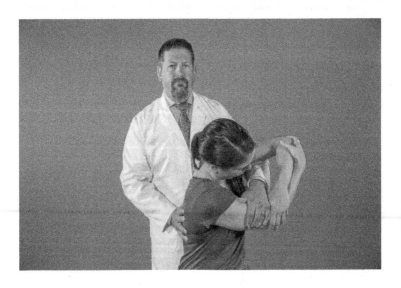

MUSCLE ENERGY—FRYETTE'S TYPE 2

1. The patient is seated.
2. Stand behind the patient.
3. Have the patient grasp his or her elbows.
4. Place your thenar eminence over the rotated side of dysfunction.
5. With your other hand, reach over the patient's folded arms and grasp the upper arm (ipsilateral to the rotation).
6. Sidebend and rotate the patient into the barrier (sidebending and rotation to the same side).
7. Have the patient gently turn his or her body back against your resisting force.
8. The patient holds the contractive force for 3 to 5 seconds and then relaxes.
9. Pause for 1 to 2 seconds.
10. Repeat steps 6 to 8 a total of three to five times.
11. Take the patient into a final stretch toward the barrier and then return the patient to neutral.
12. Reassess.

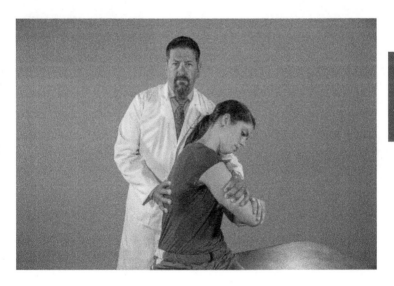

SOFT TISSUE—PERPENDICULAR STRETCH

1. The patient lies prone.
2. Stand at the side of the patient, opposite the dysfunction, and place your hands over the paravertebral musculature so that your proximal hypothenar and thenar eminences are perpendicular to the spine.
3. Apply a lateral stretch of the paravertebral musculature for about 3 seconds or until you feel the myofascial structures soften.
4. Repeat to all levels of dysfunction.
5. Reassess.

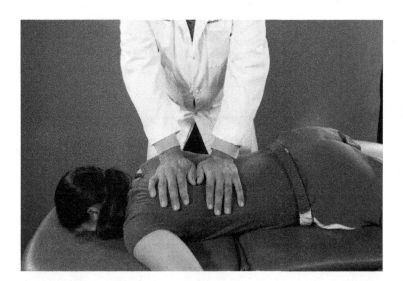

HVLA—SEATED THORACIC HVLA T1–T5 (FULL NELSON)

1. The patient is seated with his or her knees slightly extended and the back of his or her knees on the table.
2. Stand behind the patient and raise the table so that the patient's head is just below your nose.
3. Have the patient abduct his or her arms.
4. Reach your hands in front of the patient and loop your hands under his or her arms, clasping your hands over the back of the neck.
5. Have the patient clasp his or her hands over yours.
6. Lower yourself so that your sternum makes contact with the rotational component of the thoracic dysfunction to be treated. This is the fulcrum through which the corrective force is exerted.
7. Bring your elbows inward to make contact with the patient's thorax.
8. Have the patient allow his or her elbows to fall forward (but he or she should not clench).
9. Lean the patient back and quickly lift the patient posteriorly and superiorly at a 45° angle in order to impose the thrust.
10. Reassess.

Note: Be sure you are treating at the proper table height for your height.

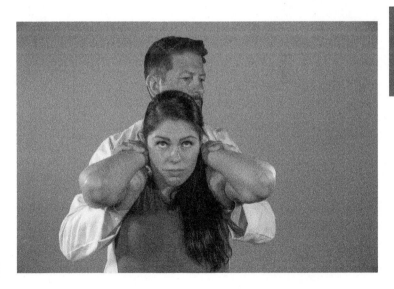

Techniques

HVLA—SUPINE DOUBLE ARM THRUST (KIRKSVILLE)

1. The patient lies supine.
2. Stand at the side of the patient, opposite the rotational dysfunction. If you have an adjustable table, lower it to the level just above your knees.
3. Cross the patient's arms over his or her chest and have him or her grasp his or her shoulders with the arm on the side of the rotational dysfunction on top.
4. Roll the patient's upper body toward you and place your thenar eminence of your caudad hand over the rotated transverse process of the segment to be treated.
5. Roll the patient's back over this hand and tuck the patient's elbows down so that the lateral aspect of the top elbow meets your epigastric region.
6. Place your cephalad hand behind the patient's head in order to flex and sidebend the upper body of the patient.
7. Make adjustments in sidebending to bring the patient to the barrier.
8. Hold the patient tightly and have the patient inhale and exhale.
9. At the end of the patient's exhalation, apply a quick downward thrust into the dysfunction (toward your caudad thenar eminence).
10. Reassess.

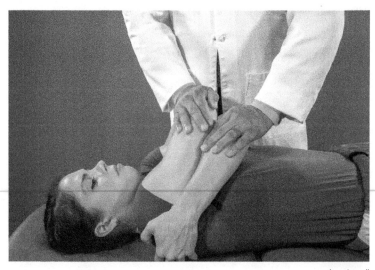

(continued)

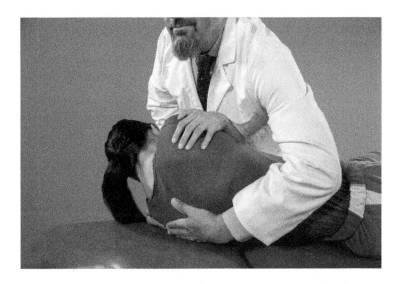

Techniques

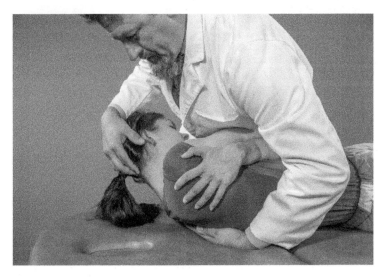

HVLA—PRONE DOUBLE ARM THRUST (TEXAS) FRYETTE'S TYPE 2

1. The patient lies prone.
2. Stand at the side of the patient on the side of the rotational component of the dysfunction and place your hypothenar eminence of caudad hand slightly inferior to the transverse processes of the area of somatic dysfunction.
3. Place the other hand slightly superior to the transverse processes of the same thoracic level on the opposite side (also opposite to the rotational component of the dysfunction).
4. To set up for the thrust, move hands in opposite directions to take up any slack of soft tissue that may be over the dysfunctional region.
5. After taking out the slack of soft tissues, your thenar/hypothenar eminences should now be over the level of the transverse process of the segment you are treating.
6. Lock your arms to maintain the force through the thrust.
7. Instruct the patient to deeply inhale and completely exhale.
8. Apply a quick anterior thrust at the very end of exhalation.
9. Reassess.

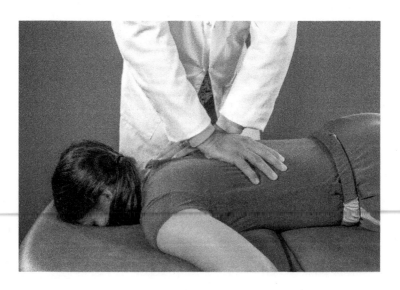

HVLA—PRONE DOUBLE ARM THRUST (TEXAS) FRYETTE'S TYPE 1

1. The patient lies prone.
2. Stand at the side of the patient on the side of the rotational component of the dysfunction and place your hypothenar eminence of cephalad hand slightly superior to the transverse processes of the area of somatic dysfunction.
3. Place the other hand slightly inferior to the transverse processes of the same thoracic level on the opposite side (also opposite to the rotational component of the dysfunction).
4. To set up for the thrust, move hands in opposite directions to take up any slack of soft tissue that may be over the dysfunctional region.
5. After taking out the slack of soft tissues, your thenar/hypothenar eminences should now be over the level of the transverse process of the segment you are treating.
6. Lock your arms to maintain the force through the thrust.
7. Instruct the patient to deeply inhale and completely exhale and apply the thrust at the very end of exhalation.
8. Reassess.

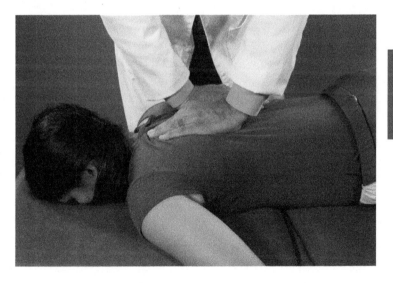

Techniques

MYOFASCIAL RELEASE DIRECT—PECTORAL TRACTION

1. The patient lies supine.
2. Stand at the head of the table and have the patient slightly abduct his or her arms.
3. Grasp the lateral aspect of the pectoral muscles and apply slow traction anteriorly and superiorly.
4. Hold for 30 seconds and release.
5. Repeat 3 to 5 times.

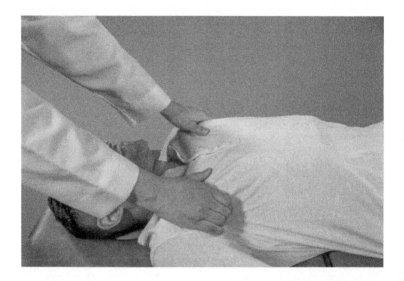

LYMPHATIC—THORACIC PUMP

1. The patient lies supine.
2. Stand at the head of the patient and have the patient slightly abduct his or her arms.
3. With your thumbs near the sternum, place the rest of your hands inferior to the clavicles and over the anterolateral aspect of ribs 2 to 5. (In female patients, push breast tissue down and away from your hands using edge of your index fingers and thumbs.)
4. Have the patient turn his or her heads to one side and take a deep breath through the mouth and then exhale.
5. As the patient exhales, exert a posterior/inferior force to exaggerate the exhalation.
6. Apply a pumping force (two pumps per second) to the thoracic cage for 3 to 5 seconds and then pause while maintaining the increased pressure on the thoracic cage.
7. Have the patient take another deep breath while resisting the motion of inhalation and then have the patient exhale.
8. Repeat steps 5 to 7 a total of three to five times.
9. After the last set of pumping forces, have the patient take another deep breath and as the patient begins to inhale, release the rib cage quickly and completely. This quick release rapidly increases the intrathoracic pressure, which can assist in the relief of atelectasis and mucous plugging.
10. Reassess rib motion.

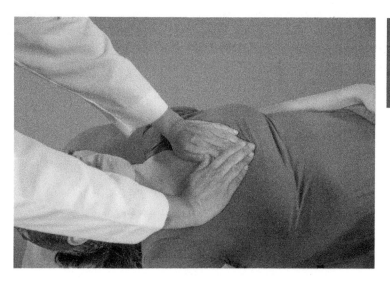

Techniques

COUNTERSTRAIN—ANTERIOR TENDERPOINTS (GENERAL)

1. The patient lies supine.
2. Stand at the side of the patient, on the same side as the dysfunction.
3. Locate the tenderpoint with your index finger (the monitoring finger must remain unmoved for the duration of the treatment).
4. Direct the patient to assign the initial tenderness as 100% to however much tenderness is felt by the patient.
5. With the patient's knees and hips flexed, rest his or her ankles on your flexed knee with your foot on the table.
6. Flexing the hips and knees to the level of the vertebrae being treated, use your caudad hand/forearm to sidebend and rotate the lumbar spine using the lower legs as levers to achieve the position of least tenderness.
7. Readjust the position to achieve the position of least tenderness with a goal of <30% of original tenderness.
8. Hold this position for 90 seconds or until a palpable release is achieved.
9. Passively return to neutral.
10. Reassess tenderpoint.

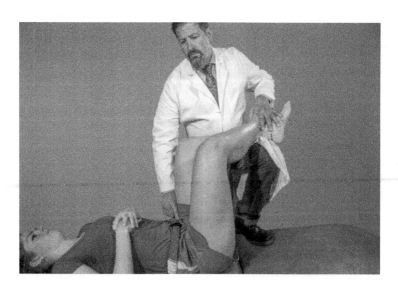

COUNTERSTRAIN—POSTERIOR TENDERPOINTS (GENERAL)

1. The patient lies prone.
2. Stand at the side of the patient, on the side opposite from the dysfunction, and locate a tenderpoint with your cephalad hand.
3. Locate the tenderpoint with your index finger (the monitoring finger must remain unmoved for the duration of the treatment).
4. Direct the patient to assign the initial tenderness as 100% to however much tenderness is felt by the patient.
5. Flex the patient's knee on the same side as the dysfunction. (Alternatively, you may stand on the side of the dysfunction and you may use your flexed knee on the table as a support for the patient's leg.)
6. With your caudad hand, cup the flexed knee.
7. Extend, abduct, and externally rotate the hip to achieve the position of least tenderness.
8. Readjust the position to achieve the position of least tenderness with a goal of <30% of original tenderness.
9. Hold this position for 90 seconds or until a palpable release is achieved.
10. Passively return to neutral.
11. Reassess tenderpoint.

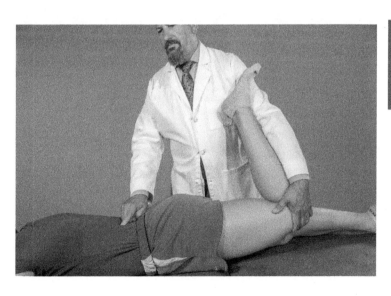

Techniques

SOFT TISSUE—PERPENDICULAR STRETCH

1. The patient lies prone.
2. Stand at the side of the patient, opposite the side of the dysfunction, and place your hand over the paravertebral musculature so that the heel of your hand (your proximal hypothenar and thenar eminences) is perpendicular to the spine.
3. Apply a lateral stretch to the paravertebral musculature for about 3 seconds and then release your pressure.
4. Repeat in a rhythmic fashion 1 to 2 minutes or until you feel the myofascial structures soften. (Alternatively, you can apply a constant lateral stretch to the paravertebral musculature for 15 to 30 seconds or until you feel the myofascial structures soften.)
5. Repeat for all levels of dysfunction.
6. Reassess.

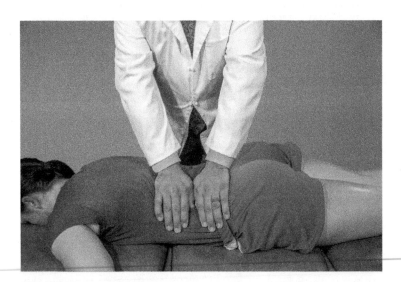

MUSCLE ENERGY—FRYETTE'S TYPE 1

1. The patient is seated.

2. Stand behind the patient.

3. Have the patient grasp his or her elbows.

4. Place your thenar eminence over the rotated side of dysfunction at the apex of the curve.

5. With your other hand, reach around to the front of the patient and under and then over the patient's folded arms.

6. Grasp the upper arm (on the side of the rotational dysfunction).

7. Have the patient flex (slump) forward to the level you are treating so that the apex of the dysfunction is under your thenar eminence (for higher dysfunctions, the patient may flex his or her head).

8. Sidebend and rotate (should be in opposite directions) the patient into the barrier.

9. Have the patient gently turn his or her body back against your resisting force (against the thenar eminence on the rotation).

10. The patient holds the contractive force for 3 to 5 seconds and then relaxes.

11. Pause for 1 to 2 seconds.

12. Take the patient further into the restrictive barrier.

13. Repeat steps 8 to 11 a total of three to five times.

14. Take the patient into a final stretch toward the barrier and then return the patient to neutral.

15. Reassess.

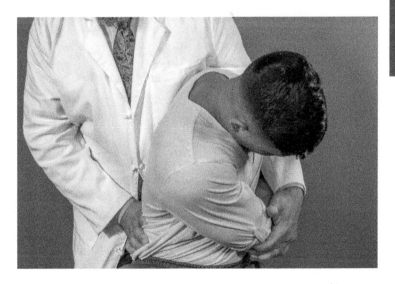

Techniques

MUSCLE ENERGY—FRYETTE'S TYPE 2

1. The patient is seated.
2. Stand behind the patient.
3. Have the patient grasp his or her elbows.
4. Place your thenar eminence over the rotated side of dysfunction.
5. With your other hand, reach over the patient's folded arms and grasp the upper arm (ipsilateral to the rotation).
6. Have the patient flex or extend into the barrier to the level you are treating.
7. Sidebend and rotate the patient into the barrier (sidebending and rotation to the same side).
8. Have the patient gently turn his or her body back against your resisting force (against the thenar eminence on the rotation).
9. The patient holds the contractive force for 3 to 5 seconds and then relaxes.
10. Pause for 1 to 2 seconds.
11. Take the patient further into the restrictive barrier.
12. Repeat steps 8 to 11 a total of three to five times.
13. Take the patient into a final stretch toward the barrier and then return the patient to neutral.
14. Reassess.

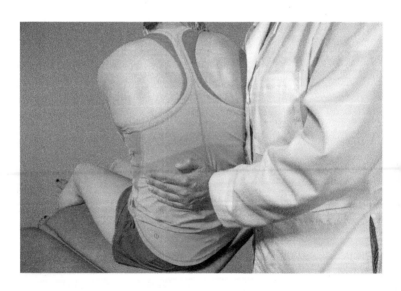

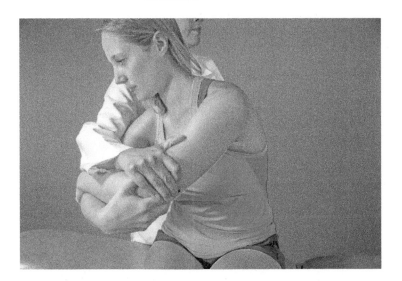

HVLA—LATERAL RECUMBENT (LUMBAR ROLL)

1. The physician stands in front of the patient.
2. The patient is in the lateral recumbent position with the rotational component of the dysfunctional side up.
3. Flex the hips and knees of the patient while monitoring the restricted vertebral segment with the cephalad hand. (More flexion will be needed to access the upper lumbar segments.)
4. Adjust until movement is palpated at the restricted segment(s).
5. Instruct the patient to extend the lower leg while maintaining the flexion of the top leg.
6. Switch hands so that your caudad hand is monitoring at the segment.
7. With your cephalad hand, pull the patient's bottom arm and turn the patient so that his or her thoracic spine is as flat on the table as physically possible for the patient (torso facing up) (figure 2).
8. Instruct the patient to grab his or her elbows with both hands.
9. Maintain the upper body positioning with the cephalad forearm by hooking your arm under the patient's folded arm and gently resting your forearm against the lateral thorax (figure 3).
10. With the caudal forearm, contact the iliac crest of the patient.
11. Rotate the patient so that all the slack of the lumbar region is taken out with torsion.
12. Instruct the patient to take a deep breath and then exhale. As the patient exhales, follow the exhalation with the caudal forearm and bring the patient to the restrictive barrier.
13. Apply the thrust by dropping your body weight through your forearm anteriorly and inferiorly.
14. Return the patient to neutral.
15. Reassess.

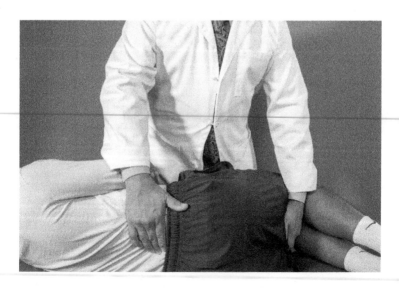

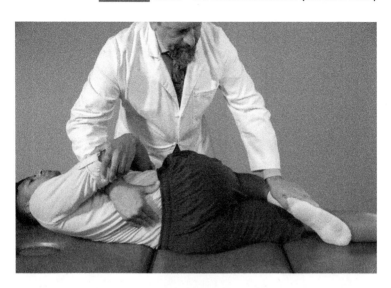

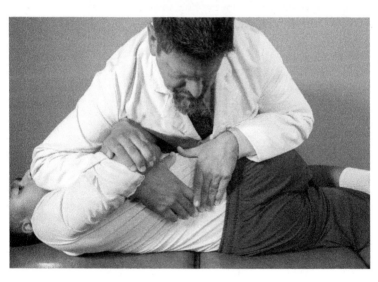

ARTICULATORY

1. The patient is supine.
2. Stand beside the patient near his or her pelvis on the side to be treated.
3. Have the patient slightly bend his or her hip and knee on the side to be treated.
4. Place your cephalad hand on the sacrum at S2.
5. With your caudad hand, grasp the leg just below the knee and flex the knee and hip to the level of S2 while palpating for motion at S2 with your opposite hand.
6. Abduct the thigh until you reach the passive barrier in abduction.
7. Add a mild compression through the knee to engage the femur into the acetabulum.
8. Externally rotate and circumduct the hip while maintaining compression.
9. Then, internally rotate and circumduct the hip also while maintaining compression.
10. Repeat steps 8 and 9 three to five times until motion improves.
11. Reassess.

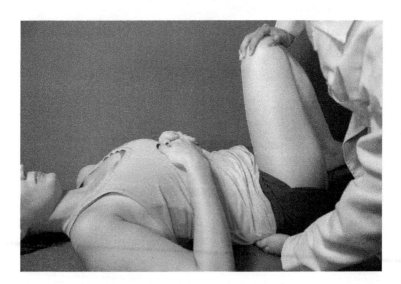

MUSCLE ENERGY—BILATERAL SACRAL FLEXION

1. The patient is prone.
2. Stand beside the patient at his or her pelvis.
3. Place the base of your palm (proximal hypothenar and thenar eminences) across the distal end of the sacrum (near the ILAs) such that your fingers are pointed toward the sacral base. Position your other hand on top of your first hand in the opposite direction. This reinforces the forces to be exerted.
4. The patient inhales and then exhales deeply.
5. As the patient inhales, follow the sacrum into counternutation.
6. As the patient exhales, resist sacral nutation by applying a gentle anterior force to the distal sacrum.
7. With each patient respiration, exaggerate counternutation during inhalation and resist nutation during exhalation.
8. Repeat steps 4 to 7 three to five times.
9. Reassess sacral motion.

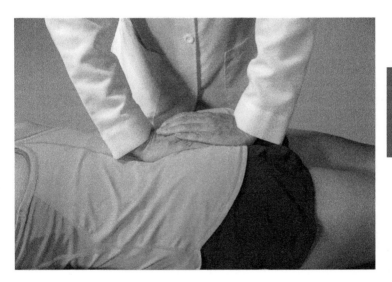

Techniques

MUSCLE ENERGY–BILATERAL EXTENSION

1. The patient is prone, preferable in the sphinx position (propped up on his or her elbows).
2. Stand beside the patient at his or her pelvis.
3. Place the base of your palm (proximal hypothenar and thenar eminences) at the sacral base such that your fingers are pointed toward the coccyx. Position your other hand on top of your first hand in the opposite direction. This reinforces the forces to be exerted.
4. The patient inhales and then exhales deeply.
5. As the patient inhales, resist sacral counternutation applying a gentle anterior force to the sacral base.
6. As the patient exhales, encourage the sacral base anteriorly into nutation by applying a gentle anterior force.
7. With each patient respiration, resist counternutation during inhalation and exaggerate nutation during exhalation.
8. Repeat steps 4 to 7 three to five times.
9. Reassess sacral motion.

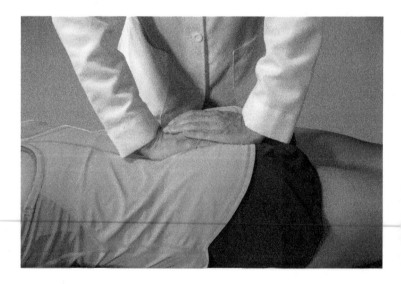

MUSCLE ENERGY—ANTERIOR TORSION

For example, right rotation on right oblique axis (R on R)
1. The patient is in a lateral recumbent position, with the axis of the dysfunction (right) facing up (off the table).
2. Stand facing the patient and have the patient flex his or her hips and knees to 90°.
3. Using the patient's right arm, turn the patient so that the torso faces upward.
4. Monitor the dysfunctional sacral base (left).
5. Raise the patient's feet toward the ceiling until the barrier is reached.
6. Instruct the patient to push toward the floor for 3 to 5 seconds, using the left gluteus maximus muscle to pull the left sacral base posteriorly and then relax.
7. Repeat steps 5 and 6 three to five times.

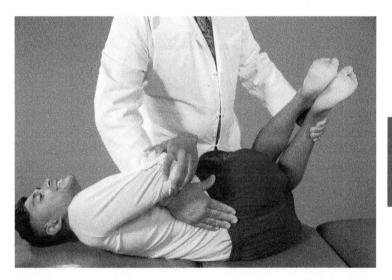

MUSCLE ENERGY—POSTERIOR TORSION

For example, right rotation on left oblique axis (R on L)

1. The patient is in a lateral recumbent position, with the axis of the dysfunction (left) facing down (on the table).
2. Have the patient lie with hips and knees flexed to 90°.
3. Stand facing the patient and, using the patient's right arm, turn the patient so that the torso faces upward.
4. Monitor the dysfunctional sacral base (right).
5. Flex the top (right) leg and hang it over the slightly less flexed left leg.
6. Push the patient's top knee toward the floor until you reach the barrier.
7. Instruct the patient to push his or her top leg toward the ceiling using the right piriformis muscle to pull the right sacral base anteriorly for 3 to 5 seconds and then relax.
8. Repeat steps 6 and 7 three to five times.

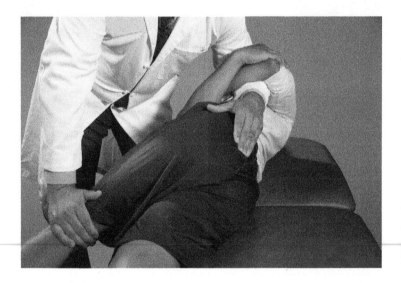

MUSCLE ENERGY JOINT MOBILIZATION—ANTERIOR INNOMINATE ROTATION DYSFUNCTION

1. The patient lies supine.
2. Stand at the side of the patient and flex the hip and knee on the side of the dysfunction.
3. Place one hand posterior to the SI joint to monitor and pull PSIS inferiorly.
4. Contact the knee of the patient and flex the hip until an innominate rotation restrictive barrier is contacted.
5. Instruct the patient to push back against you (using hamstring muscle and gluteus muscle) while you maintain an equal opposing force for 3 to 5 seconds.
6. Instruct the patient to relax.
7. After 1 second, rotate the patient's innominate further to contact the next restrictive barrier.
8. Repeat 3 to 5 times.
9. Return to neutral.
10. Reassess.

Alternate setup: You can use more of your own body weight instead of upper body strength by placing the flexed leg over your shoulder and leaning forward further as the restrictive barriers are contacted.

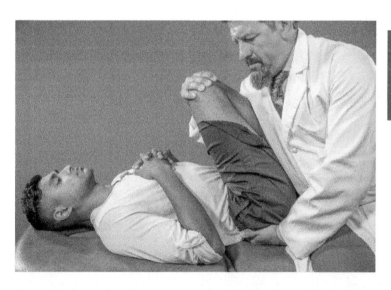

MUSCLE ENERGY JOINT MOBILIZATION—POSTERIOR INNOMINATE ROTATION DYSFUNCTION: PATIENT SUPINE

1. The patient lies supine and as close to the edge of the table as possible.
2. Stand at the side of the table, on the same side of the dysfunction, and stabilize the patient by holding him or her at the contralateral ASIS.
3. On the side of dysfunction, drop the patient's leg off the side of the table in order to extend the hip. (Be sure the table height is adequate to keep the patient's foot from hitting the floor.)
4. Contact the patient's knee and extend the hip, rotating the innominate posteriorly into its barrier.
5. Instruct the patient to push his or her knee up (anteriorly) against you (using rectus femoris of the quadriceps, sartorius, and iliacus) while you maintain an equal opposing force for 3 to 5 seconds.
6. Instruct the patient to relax.
7. Extend the patient's hip further, rotating the innominate anterior to contact the next restrictive barrier.
8. Repeat steps 4 to 6 three to five times.
9. Return to neutral.
10. Reassess.

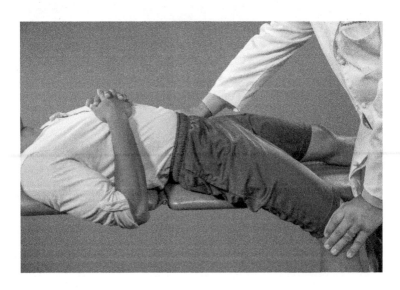

MUSCLE ENERGY JOINT MOBILIZATION—POSTERIOR INNOMINATE ROTATION DYSFUNCTION: ALTERNATE PRONE SETUP

1. The patient lies prone.
2. Stand at the side of the patient, on the side opposite the dysfunction, and have the patient flex the knee on the side of the dysfunction.
3. Place your caudad hand under the knee and extend the hip, anteriorly rotating the innominate to the restrictive barrier.
4. Ask the patient to push the dysfunctional knee down toward the table for 3 to 5 seconds.
5. Instruct the patient to relax.
6. Extend the patient's hip further to contact the next innominate rotational restrictive barrier.
7. Repeat steps 4 to 6 three to five times.
8. Return to neutral.
9. Reassess.

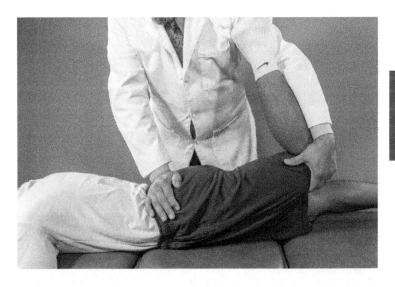

Techniques

MUSCLE ENERGY JOINT MOBILIZATION—INFLARE DYSFUNCTION

1. The patient lies supine.

2. Stand at the side of the patient on the same side as the dysfunctional innominate.

3. The leg of the dysfunctional side is positioned with the knee and hip flexed and the hip externally rotated and abducted into a figure "4" position.

4. Place one of your hands on the ASIS of the contralateral side. (This placement is for stabilization of the pelvis during the treatment.)

5. Place your other hand on the knee of the dysfunctional side.

6. Apply a force on the contacted knee until the restrictive barrier is felt.

7. Instruct the patient to push his or her knee anteriorly against your resistive force (engaging adductor muscles).

8. Hold the position for 3 to 5 seconds.

9. Instruct the patient to relax.

10. Repeat steps 6 to 9 three to five times, always bringing the patient to the new barrier.

11. Bring the leg back to neutral.

12. Reassess.

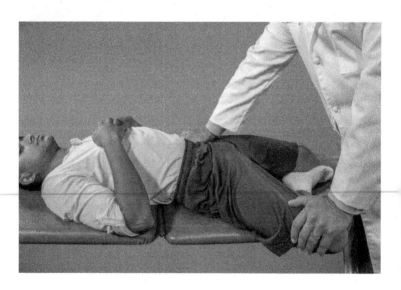

MUSCLE ENERGY JOINT MOBILIZATION—OUTFLARE DYSFUNCTION

1. The patient lies supine.
2. Stand at the side of the patient, on the same side as the dysfunction.
3. Flex the patient's knee and hip to 90°.
4. Place patient's foot on table and adduct and internally rotate hip across the patient's midline.
5. With one hand, reach under patient and apply lateral traction at posterior superior iliac spine of the dysfunctional side.
6. Instruct the patient to push hip back against you trying to externally rotate and abduct the leg (contracting the gluteus maximus muscle). Apply counterforce for 3 to 5 seconds.
7. Instruct the patient to relax.
8. After 1 second, bring the patient to the new barrier.
9. Repeat steps 6 to 8 three to five times.
10. Bring the leg back to neutral.
11. Reassess.

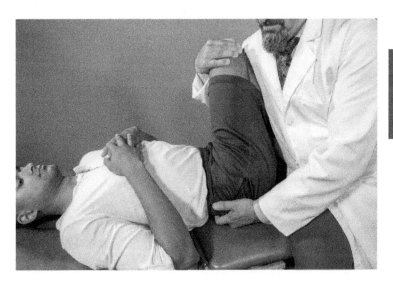

Techniques

MUSCLE ENERGY JOINT MOBILIZATION/RESPIRATORY ASSIST—SUPERIOR INNOMINATE SHEAR DYSFUNCTION

1. The patient lies supine.
2. Stand at the end of the table by the patient's feet.
3. Brace the patient's foot of the leg opposite of the dysfunction on your thigh.
4. Pick up the leg on the side of the dysfunction to approximately 10 inches off of the table and securely hold foot and ankle. Internally rotate and slightly abduct the hip.
5. Instruct the patient to take deep breaths as you apply traction down the length of the leg.
6. Take up any slack as the patient exhale. [1]A quick tug after the last breath is often added as an HVLA technique.
7. Repeat steps 5 and 6 three to five times.
8. Return to neutral.
9. Reassess.

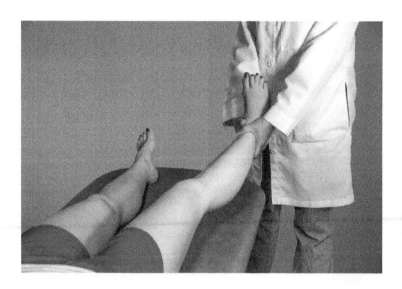

MUSCLE ENERGY JOINT MOBILIZATION/RESPIRATORY ASSIST—INFERIOR INNOMINATE SHEAR DYSFUNCTION

1. The patient lies supine.
2. Stand at the end of the table by the patient's feet.
3. Brace the patient's foot of the leg on the side of the dysfunction on your thigh. (This treatment pushes the innominate superiorly using the leg resting on your thigh.)
4. Pick up the leg on the side opposite of the dysfunction to approximately 10 inches off of the table and securely hold foot and ankle. Internally rotate and slightly abduct the hip.
5. Instruct the patient to take deep breaths as you apply traction down the length of the leg.
6. Take up any slack as the patient exhale.
7. Repeat steps 5 and 6 three to five times.
8. Return to neutral.
9. Reassess.

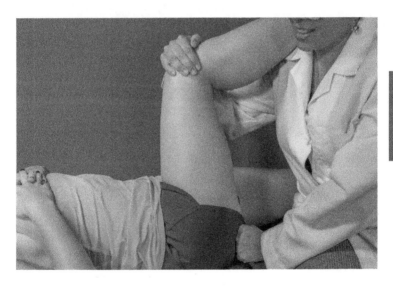

Techniques

213

CARPAL BONE—ARTICULATORY

1. The patient is seated.
2. Sit facing the patient at eye level.
3. The patient's elbow is flexed such that his or her fingers are facing superiorly and anteriorly.
4. Place the heels of your hands over both sides of the patient's wrist, covering the patient's carpal bones. Interlace your fingers.
5. Add mild compression and distraction superiorly and anteriorly.
6. Circumduct the wrist clockwise and counterclockwise (through flexion, adduction, extension, and abduction) for 15 to 30 seconds to mobilize the carpal bones.
7. Reassess.

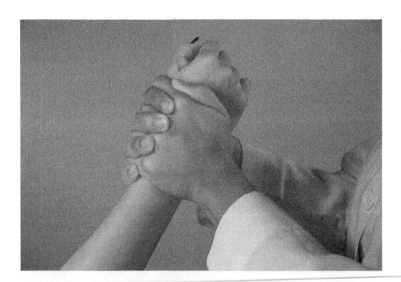

FLEXOR RETINACULUM RELEASE (CARPAL TUNNEL TREATMENT)—MYOFASCIAL RELEASE

1. The patient is seated.
2. Stand or sit in front of the patient.
3. The patient's hand and wrist are supine.
4. Place your thumbs on the midline of the flexor retinaculum (center wrist) and your curled fingers are securing the dorsal side of the patient's hand.
5. Slightly extend the patient's wrist.
6. Without sliding over the skin, separate your thumbs to add lateral tension to the skin and superficial fascia with the thumbs.
7. Apply this tension for 15 to 30 seconds or until a release of tissue tension is palpated. Repeat 3 to 5 times if needed.
8. Reassess.

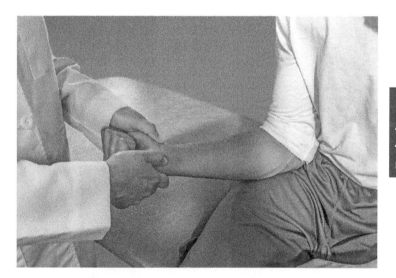

Techniques

SPENCER TECHNIQUE—ARTICULATORY

Initial positioning
1. The patient is in a lateral recumbent position, with the shoulder to be treated up, away from the table, and the elbow flexed.
2. Stand facing the patient at the level of the shoulder.
3. Your cephalad hand bridges the shoulder, locking out any acromioclavicular and scapulothoracic motion by placing your fingers on the spine of the scapula and your thumb on the clavicle.
4. With your caudad hand, grasp the patient's forearm.

Stage 1 extension
5. Move the patient's shoulder into extension to the restrictive barrier (or anatomical barrier). If there is a restrictive barrier, apply a slow, gentle, springing motion toward extension.
6. Switch hands so that your caudad hand reaches over and behind the patient. The fingers of your caudad hand are on the clavicle, and the heels of your hand (proximal hypothenar and thenar eminences) are on the spine of the scapula.

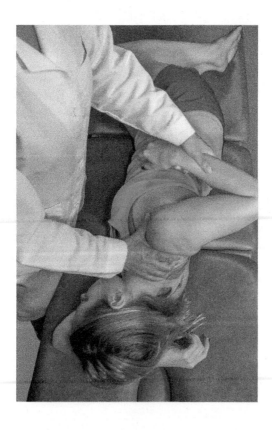

Stage 2 flexion

7. With the elbow in extension, bring the shoulder into flexion to the restrictive barrier (or anatomical barrier).
   - If there is a restrictive barrier, apply a slow, gentle, springing motion toward flexion.
8. Switch back to the original hand placement. Your cephalad hand bridges the shoulder, locking out any acromioclavicular and scapulothoracic motion by placing your fingers on the spine of the scapula and your thumb on the clavicle.

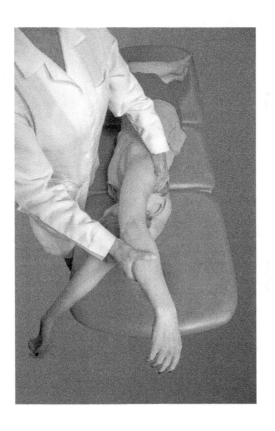

Techniques

Stage 3a circumduction: compression

9. With your caudad hand, cup the flexed elbow and abduct the shoulder to 90°, move the elbow in small clockwise circles with compression into the glenohumeral joint. Repeat in the opposite direction for a total of 15 to 30 seconds.

- If there is a restrictive barrier, the circumduction and compression would help to remove restrictions.

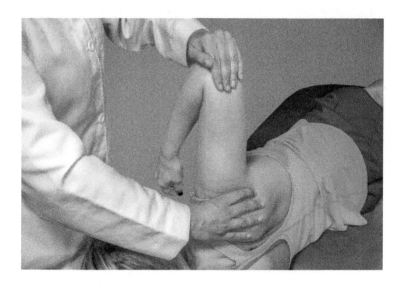

Stage 3b circumduction: traction

10. With the arm still abducted to 90°, extend the elbow and add traction with circumduction using larger clockwise circles with traction and then in the opposite direction for a total of 15 to 30 seconds.

- If there is a restrictive barrier, the circumduction and traction would help to remove restrictions.

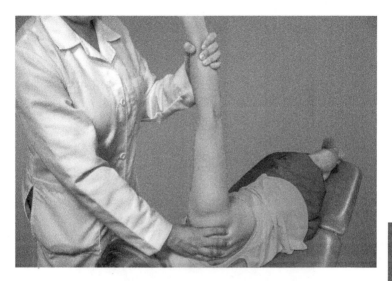

Stage 4 abduction

11. Rest the patient's hand on your cephalad forearm.
12. Lift the elbow laterally, taking the shoulder into abduction to the restrictive barrier (or anatomical barrier).
    - If there is a restrictive barrier, apply a slow, gentle, springing motion on the elbow toward abduction of the shoulder.

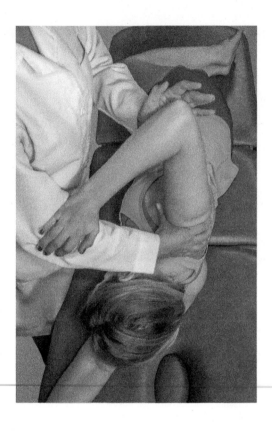

Stage 5 adduction and external rotation
13. Move the elbow medially, taking the shoulder into adduction and external rotation to the restrictive barrier (or anatomical barrier).
- If there is a restrictive barrier, apply a slow, gentle, springing motion on the elbow toward adduction and external rotation of the shoulder.

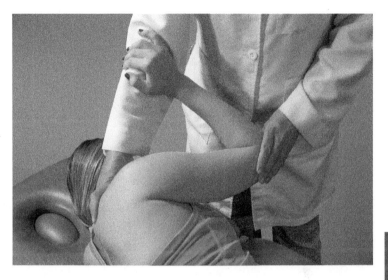

Techniques

Stage 6 internal rotation

14. Ask the patient to put his or her wrist and hand behind the back.
15. Gently pull the elbow anteriorly to its restrictive barrier (or anatomical barrier) to test for internal rotation.
   • If there is a restrictive barrier, apply a slow, gentle, springing motion on the elbow toward internal rotation of the shoulder.

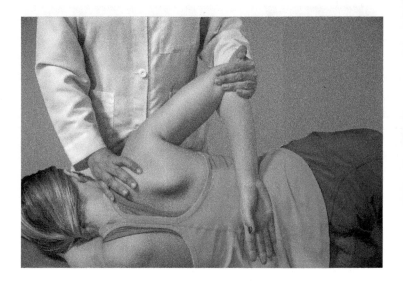

Stage 7 deltoid muscle pump

16. Rest the patient's hand on your caudad shoulder.

17. With your interlaced fingers, cup the posterior aspect of the deltoid muscle and repeatedly draw the proximal humerus anteriorly (pumping motion).

  • If there is a restrictive barrier, the pumping motion would help to remove restrictions.

18. Reasses

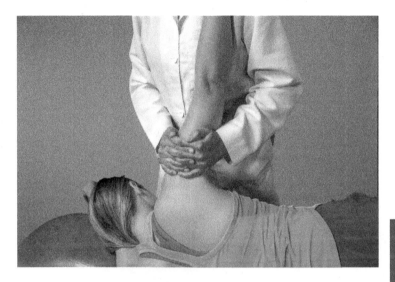

SPENCER TECHNIQUE—MUSCLE ENERGY

Initial positioning

1. The patient is in a lateral recumbent position, with the shoulder to be treated up, away from the table and his or her elbow flexed.
2. Stand facing the patient at the level of the shoulder.
3. Your cephalad hand bridges the shoulder, locking out any acromioclavicular and scapulothoracic motion by placing your fingers on the spine of the scapula and your thumb on the clavicle.
4. With your caudad hand, grasp the patient's forearm.

Stage 1 extension

5. Move the patient's shoulder into extension to the restrictive barrier (or anatomical barrier).
   a. If there is a restrictive barrier, instruct the patient to move his or her shoulder toward flexion against your resistance.
   b. Hold for 3 to 5 seconds and then ask the patient to relax.
   c. Take the patient to the next barrier toward extension.
   d. Repeat steps b and c three to five times.
   e. Apply a final stretch toward the barrier.
   f. Reassess.
6. Switch hands so that your caudad hand reaches over and behind the patient. The fingers of your caudad hand are on the clavicle, and the heels of your hand (proximal hypothenar and thenar eminences) are on the spine of the scapula.

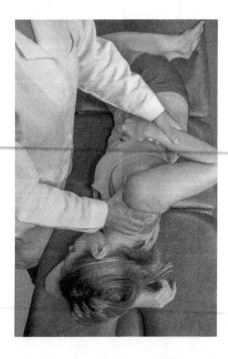

Stage 2 flexion

7. With the elbow in extension, bring the shoulder into flexion to the restrictive barrier (or anatomical barrier).

   a. If there is a restrictive barrier, instruct the patient to move his or her shoulder toward extension against your resistance.

   b. Hold for 3 to 5 seconds and then ask the patient to relax.

   c. Take the patient to the next barrier toward flexion.

   d. Repeat steps b and c three to five times.

   e. Apply a final stretch toward the barrier.

   f. Reassess.

8. Switch back to the original hand placement. Your cephalad hand bridges the shoulder, locking out any acromioclavicular and scapulothoracic motion by placing your fingers on the spine of the scapula and your thumb on the clavicle.

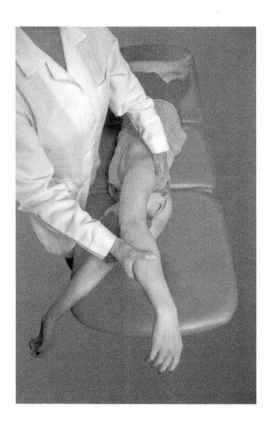

Techniques

Stage 3a circumduction: compression

9. With your caudad hand, cup the flexed elbow and abduct the shoulder to 90°, move the elbow in small clockwise circles with compression into the glenohumeral joint. Repeat in the opposite direction for a total of 15 to 30 seconds.

- If there is a restrictive barrier, the circumduction and compression would help to remove restrictions (there is no MET version for this stage).

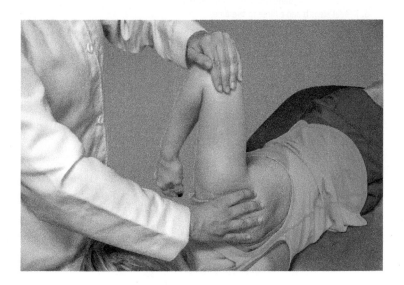

Stage 3b circumduction: traction

10. With the arm still abducted to 90°, extend the elbow and add traction with circumduction, using larger clockwise circles with traction and then in the opposite direction for a total of 15 to 30 seconds.

- If there is a restrictive barrier, the circumduction and traction would help to remove restrictions (there is no MET version for this stage).

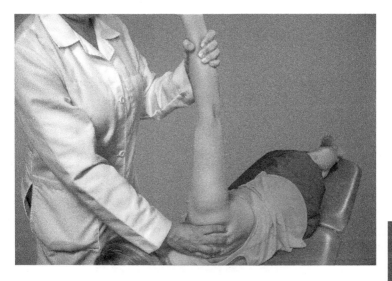

Stage 4 abduction

11. Rest the patient's hand on your cephalad forearm.
12. Lift the elbow laterally, taking the shoulder into abduction to the restrictive barrier (or anatomical barrier).
    a. If there is a restrictive barrier, instruct the patient to move his or her elbow medially toward adduction against your resistance.
    b. Hold for 3 to 5 seconds and then ask the patient to relax.
    c. Take the patient to the next barrier toward abduction.
    d. Repeat steps b and c three to five times.
    e. Apply a final stretch toward the barrier.
    f. Reassess.

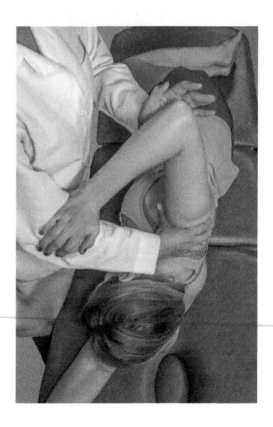

Stage 5 adduction and external rotation

13. Move the elbow medially, taking the shoulder into adduction and externally rotate to the restrictive barrier (or anatomical barrier).

   a. If there is a restrictive barrier, instruct the patient to move his or her elbow laterally toward abduction against your resistance.

   b. Hold for 3 to 5 seconds and then ask the patient to relax.

   c. Take the patient to the next barrier toward adduction.

   d. Repeat steps b and c three to five times.

   e. Apply a final stretch toward the barrier.

   f. Reassess.

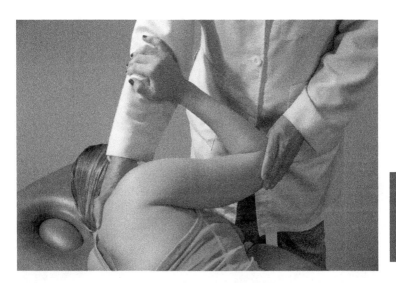

Stage 6 internal rotation

14. Ask the patient to put his or her wrist and hand behind his or her back.
15. Gently pull the elbow anteriorly to its restrictive barrier (or anatomical barrier) to test for internal rotation.
    a. If there is a restrictive barrier, instruct the patient to move his or her elbow posteriorly toward external rotation against your resistance.
    b. Hold for 3 to 5 seconds and then ask the patient to relax.
    c. Take the patient to the next barrier toward internal rotation.
    d. Repeat steps b and c three to five times.
    e. Apply a final stretch toward the barrier.
    f. Reassess.

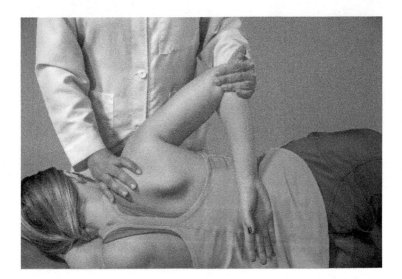

Stage 7 deltoid muscle pump

16. Rest the patient's hand on your caudad shoulder.

17. With interlaced fingers, cup the posterior aspect of the deltoid muscle and repeatedly draw the proximal humerus anteriorly (pumping motion).

- If there is a restrictive barrier, the pumping motion would help to remove restrictions (there is no MET version for this stage).

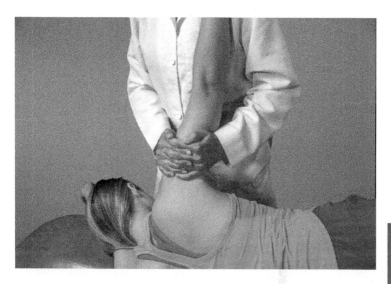

Techniques

COUNTERSTRAIN—SUPRASPINATUS

1. The patient lies supine.
2. Sit beside the patient, on the same side as the dysfunction at the level of the shoulder.
3. Locate a tenderpoint in the belly of the supraspinatus muscle with the index finger of your cephalad hand (the monitoring finger must remain unmoved for the duration of the treatment).
4. Direct the patient to assign the initial tenderness as 100% to however much tenderness is felt by the patient.
5. Flex and abduct the shoulder with marked external rotation to achieve the position of least tenderness with a goal of <30% of original tenderness.
6. Hold for 90 seconds or until a release is felt.
7. Passively return to neutral.
8. Reassess tenderpoint.

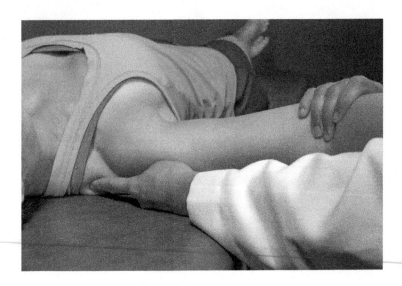

COUNTERSTRAIN—INFRASPINATUS

1. The patient lies supine.
2. Sit beside the patient, on the same side as the dysfunction at the level of the shoulder.
3. With the index finger of your cephalad hand, locate a tenderpoint which is inferior and lateral to the spine of the scapula at the posterior medial aspect of the glenohumeral joint (the monitoring finger must remain unmoved for the duration of the treatment).
4. Direct the patient to assign the initial tenderness as 100% to however much tenderness is felt by the patient.
5. Flex the shoulder to 90° to 120° and abduct the shoulder as well to achieve the position of least tenderness with a goal of <30% of original tenderness.
6. You may add internal and external rotation as needed.
7. Hold for 90 seconds or until a release is felt.
8. Passively return to neutral.
9. Reassess tenderpoint.

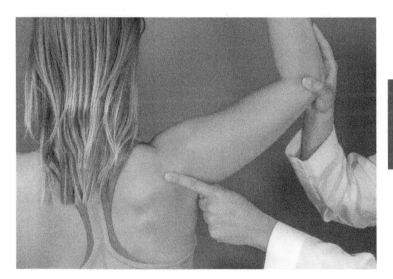

COUNTERSTRAIN—TERES MAJOR

1. The patient lies supine with the shoulder slightly off the edge of the table.
2. Sit beside the patient, on the same side as the dysfunction at the level of the shoulder.
3. With the index finger of your cephalad hand, locate the tenderpoint on the posterior lateral surface on the inferior border of the scapula (the monitoring finger must remain unmoved for the duration of the treatment).
4. Direct the patient to assign the initial tenderness as 100% to however much tenderness is felt by the patient.
5. Extend the shoulder to 30° and flex the elbow to 90°.
6. Significantly, internally rotate the shoulder to achieve the position of least tenderness with a goal of <30% of original tenderness.
7. Hold for 90 seconds or until a release is felt.
8. Passively return to neutral.
9. Reassess tenderpoint.

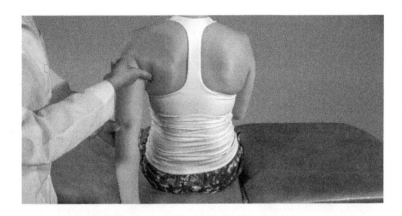

COUNTERSTRAIN—TERES MINOR

1. The patient lies supine with the shoulder slightly off the edge of the table.

2. Sit beside the patient, on the same side as the dysfunction at the level of the shoulder.

3. With the index finger of your cephalad hand, locate the tenderpoint in the lateral border of the upper scapula (the monitoring finger must remain unmoved for the duration of the treatment).

4. Direct the patient to assign the initial tenderness as 100% to however much tenderness is felt by the patient.

5. Extend the arm with slight adduction and significant external rotation of the shoulder to achieve the position of least tenderness with a goal of <30% of original tenderness.

6. Hold for 90 seconds or until a release is felt.

7. Passively return to neutral.

8. Reassess tenderpoint.

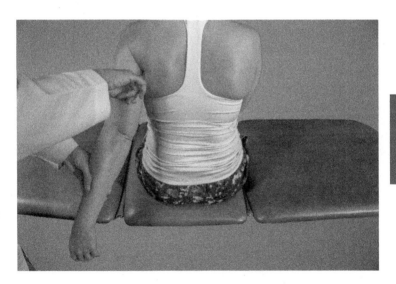

COUNTERSTRAIN—SUBSCAPULARIS

1. The patient lies supine, with the shoulder slightly off the edge of the table.
2. Sit beside the patient, on the same side as the dysfunction at the level of the shoulder.
3. With the index finger of your cephalad hand, locate the tenderpoint in the posterior axilla, at the anterolateral border of the scapula on the subscapularis muscle (the monitoring finger must remain unmoved for the duration of the treatment).
4. Direct the patient to assign the initial tenderness as 100% to however much tenderness is felt by the patient.
5. Extend and internally rotate the shoulder to achieve the position of least tenderness with a goal of <30% of original tenderness.
6. Hold for 90 seconds or until a release is felt.
7. Passively return to neutral.
8. Reassess tenderpoint.

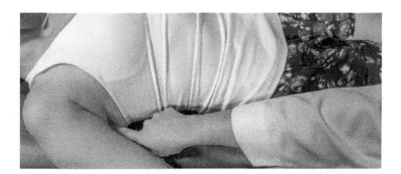

COUNTERSTRAIN—COMMON FLEXORS OF THE WRIST

1. The patient lies supine.
2. Sit beside the patient, on the same side as the dysfunction at the level of the shoulder.
3. With the index finger of your cephalad hand, locate the tenderpoint on the medial epicondyle of the humerus at the common flexor tendon (the monitoring finger must remain unmoved for the duration of the treatment).
4. Direct the patient to assign the initial tenderness as 100% to however much tenderness is felt by the patient.
5. Flex, pronate, and adduct the forearm while slightly flexing the wrist to achieve the position of least tenderness with a goal of <30% of original tenderness.
6. Hold for 90 seconds or until a release is felt.
7. Passively return to neutral.
8. Reassess tenderpoint.

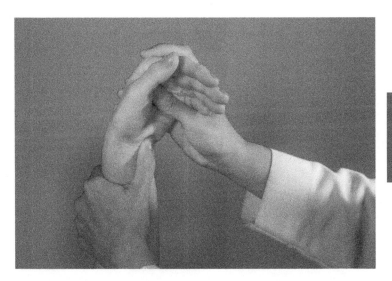

Techniques

COUNTERSTRAIN—COMMON EXTENSORS OF THE WRIST

1. The patient lies supine.
2. Sit beside the patient, on the same side as the dysfunction at the level of the shoulder.
3. With the index finger of your cephalad hand, locate the tenderpoint on the anterolateral aspect of the radial head at the common extensor tendon (the monitoring finger must remain unmoved for the duration of the treatment).
4. Direct the patient to assign the initial tenderness as 100% to however much tenderness is felt by the patient.
5. Extend the elbow and supinate the forearm to achieve the position of least tenderness with a goal of <30% of original tenderness.
6. Hold for 90 seconds or until a release is felt.
7. Passively return to neutral.
8. Reassess tenderpoint.

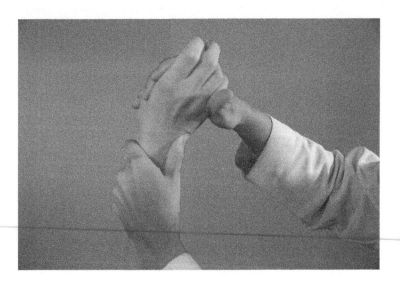

LYMPHATIC—EFFLEURAGE

1. The patient lies in the lateral recumbent position with the dysfunctional side up.
2. Stand facing the patient and encircle the patient's arm with your hands at the most proximal portion where edema is present.
3. Apply a gentle stroking motion of the soft tissue toward the shoulder.
4. Repeat this motion starting more distally with each stroke until the end of the edematous area is reached.

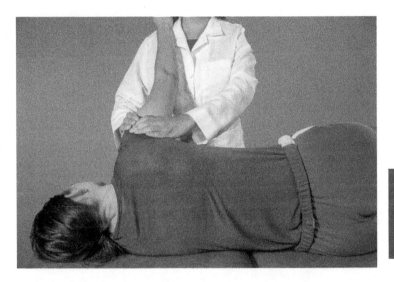

Techniques

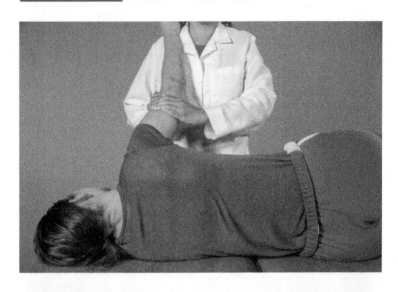

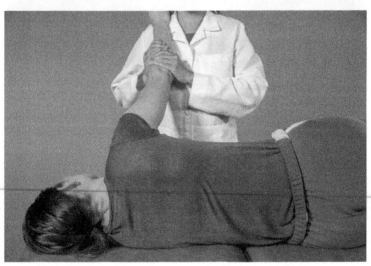

MUSCLE ENERGY—POSTERIOR RADIAL HEAD DYSFUNCTION (PRONATION DYSFUNCTION)

1. The patient is seated.
2. Stand at the side of the patient, on the side of the dysfunction, and take the patient's hand in a handshake grip and then grasp the patient's elbow with your other hand.
3. With your thumb at the elbow, apply an anterior pressure over the proximal radial head.
4. Take the patient's forearm into supination with your handshake grip hand until you reach the barrier.
5. Instruct the patient to turn the forearm toward pronation against your resistance (using pronator teres muscle).
6. Hold for 3 to 5 seconds and then ask the patient to relax.
7. Take the patient to the next barrier.
8. Repeat steps 5 to 7 three to five times.

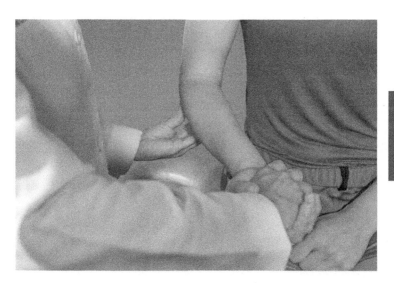

MUSCLE ENERGY—ANTERIOR RADIAL HEAD DYSFUNCTION (SUPINATION DYSFUNCTION)

1. The patient is seated.
2. Stand at the side of the patient, on the side of the dysfunction, and take the patient into a handshake grip and then grasp the patient's elbow with your other hand.
3. With your thumb, apply a posterior pressure over the proximal radial head.
4. Take the patient's forearm into pronation with your handshake grip hand until you reach the barrier.
5. Instruct the patient to turn his or her forearm toward supination against your resistance (using the supinator muscle and biceps brachii).
6. Hold for 3 to 5 seconds and then ask the patient to relax.
7. Take the patient to the next barrier.
8. Repeat steps 5 to 7 three to five times.

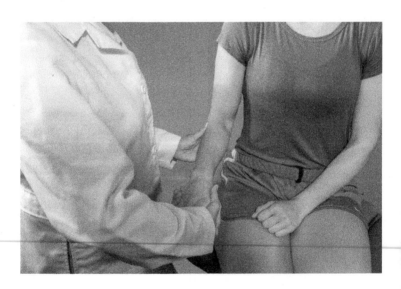

LYMPHATIC PEDAL PUMP

1. The patient lies supine.
2. Stand at the foot of the table and completely dorsiflex both of the patient's feet with your hands.
3. Without losing any of the dorsiflexion, apply a pumping force (two pumps per second) to the soles of the feet so that the entire body of the patient moves.
4. Continue for 3 to 5 minutes.

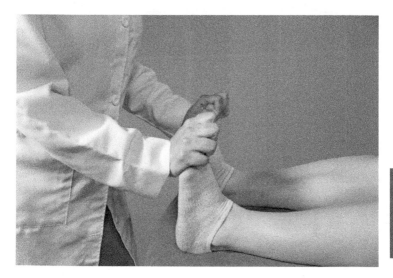

LYMPHATIC—EFFLEURAGE

1. The patient lies supine.
2. The physician sits next to the patient on the side of the dysfunction.
3. Apply a gentle stroking motion of the soft tissue toward the pelvis.
4. Repeat this motion starting more distally with each stroke until the end of the edematous area is reached.

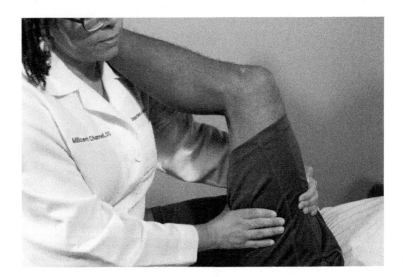

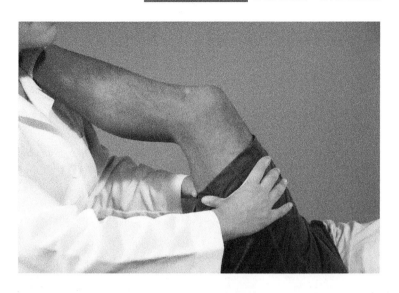

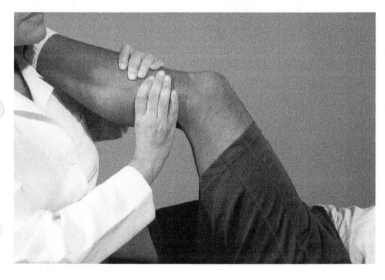

MUSCLE ENERGY—PSOAS HYPERTONICITY

1. The patient lies prone.
2. Stand at the side of the patient, on the opposite side of the dysfunction, and ask the patient to flex the knee on the side of the dysfunction.
3. Place your cephalad hand on the paraspinals at T12–L2 and cup the patient's bent knee with your caudad hand.
4. Extend the patient's hip to the restrictive barrier.
5. Have the patient isometrically contract the psoas muscle, attempting to lower the leg to the table, for 3 to 5 seconds and then ask the patient to relax and take the patient to the next barrier.
6. Repeat steps 4 and 5 three to five times.

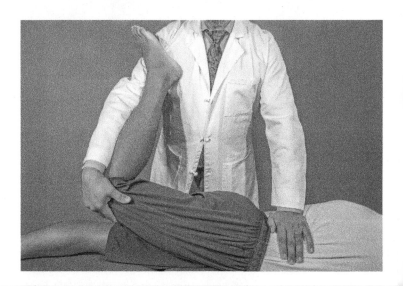

MUSCLE ENERGY—PIRIFORMIS HYPERTONICITY

1. The patient lies supine.
2. Stand or sit at the side of the patient, on the side of the dysfunction, and ask the patient to flex the knee and hip on the side of the dysfunction.
3. Internally rotate the patient's hip to the restrictive barrier.
4. Have the patient isometrically contract the piriformis, attempting to externally rotate the hip, for 3 to 5 seconds.
5. Instruct the patient to relax and take the patient to the next barrier.
6. Repeat 3 to 5 times.

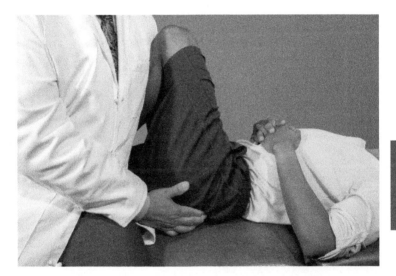

Techniques

COUNTERSTRAIN—PSOAS HYPERTONICITY

1. The patient lies supine.
2. Stand at the side of the patient, on the side of the dysfunction.
3. Locate the tenderpoint with your index finger (the monitoring finger must remain unmoved for the duration of the treatment).
4. Direct the patient to assign the initial tenderness as 100% to however much tenderness is felt by the patient.
5. Passively flex the knee and hip to find a position that decreases the tenderness at the tenderpoint.
6. Readjust the position to achieve the position of least tenderness with a goal of <30% of original tenderness.
7. Hold this position for 90 seconds or until a palpable release is achieved.
8. Passively return to neutral.
9. Reassess tenderpoint.

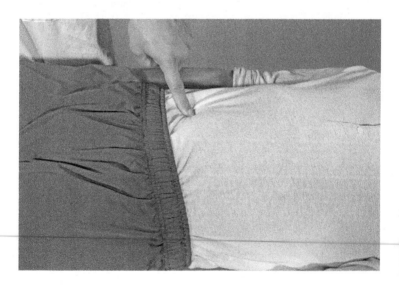

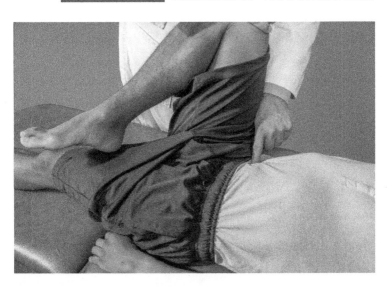

COUNTERSTRAIN—PIRIFORMIS HYPERTONICITY

1. The patient lies supine.
2. Stand or sit at the side of the patient, on the side of the dysfunction.
3. Locate the tenderpoint with your index finger (the monitoring finger must remain unmoved for the duration of the treatment).
4. Direct the patient to assign the initial tenderness as 100% to however much tenderness is felt by the patient.
5. Passively flex the knee and externally rotate the hip to find a position that decreases the tenderness at the tenderpoint.
6. Readjust the position to achieve the position of least tenderness with a goal of <30% of original tenderness.
7. Hold this position for 90 seconds or until a palpable release is achieved.
8. Passively return to neutral.
9. Reassess tenderpoint.

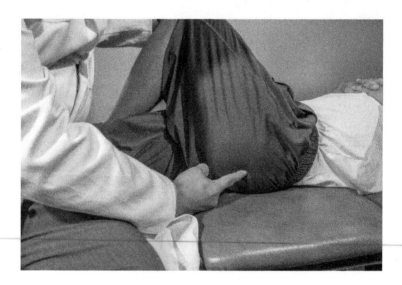

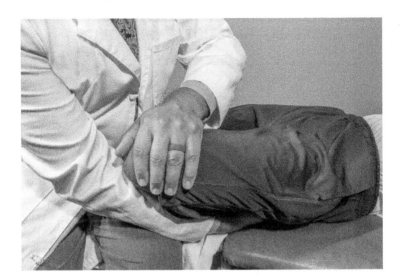

COUNTERSTRAIN—ANTERIOR TENDERPOINTS AR1–AR10

1. The patient lies supine or may be seated.
2. Stand behind the patient and identify the most tender anterior tenderpoint.
3. Locate the anterior tenderpoint with your index finger (the monitoring finger must remain unmoved for the duration of the treatment).
4. Direct the patient to assign the initial tenderness as 100% to however much tenderness is felt by the patient.
5. Use the opposite hand to position the patient into flexion, sidebending toward and rotation toward the tenderpoint. (This may be accomplished with your leg on the table resting the patient's arm on the side opposite of the tenderpoint over your knee. Placing the patient's legs on the table on the side of the tenderpoint may also be beneficial.)
6. Readjust the position to achieve the position of least tenderness with a goal of <30% of original tenderness.
7. Hold this position for 90 seconds or until a palpable release is achieved.
8. Passively return patient back to neutral position without the help of the patient.
9. Reassess for tenderness.

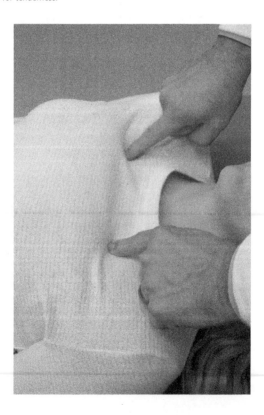

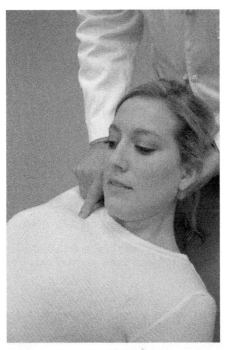

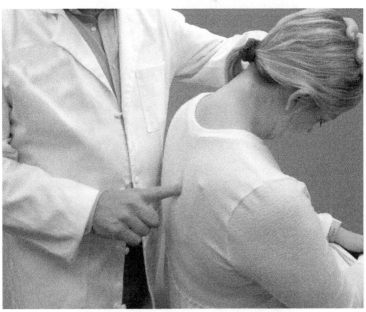

COUNTERSTRAIN—POSTERIOR TENDERPOINTS PR1–PR10

1. The patient is seated.
2. Stand behind the patient and identify the most tender posterior tenderpoint.
3. Locate the posterior tenderpoint with your index finger (the monitoring finger must remain unmoved for the duration of the treatment).
4. Direct the patient to assign the initial tenderness as 100% to however much tenderness is felt by the patient.
5. Use the opposite hand to position the patient into extension (PR1) or flexion (PR2–PR10), sidebending and rotating away from (toward for PR1) the tenderpoint. (This may be accomplished with your leg on the table resting the patient's arm on the side of the tenderpoint over your knee. Placing the patient's legs on the table on the side of the tenderpoint may also be beneficial.)
6. Readjust the position to achieve the position of least tenderness with a goal of <30% of original tenderness.
7. Hold this position for 90 seconds or until a palpable release is achieved.
8. Passively return patient back to neutral position without the help of the patient.
9. Reassess for tenderness.

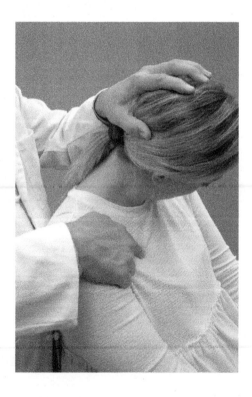

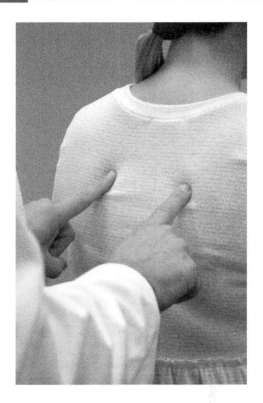

Techniques

SPRINGING TECHNIQUE (MYOFASCIAL RELEASE)—RIB RAISING

1. The patient lies supine.
2. Sit at the side of the patient and place the finger pads of both of your hands under the patient at the level of ribs to be treated approximately 2 inches from the spinous processes (just lateral to the transverse processes).
3. Lift anteriorly and then laterally by levering your forearms against the table.
4. Lower your arms back to the patient's original position.
5. Repeat for approximately 2 to 3 minutes or until there is a release and better rib motion.

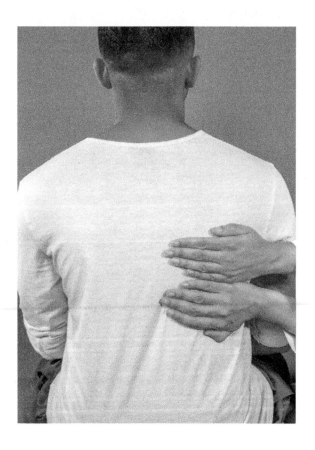

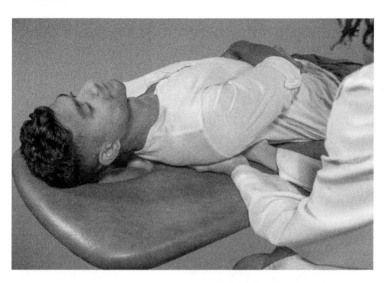

MUSCLE ENERGY USING RESPIRATORY ASSIST—FIRST OR SECOND RIB INHALATION DYSFUNCTION

1. The patient lies supine.
2. Stand at the head of the patient, holding the patient's head in one hand while contacting the lateral aspect of the dysfunctional rib with the other thumb.
3. Instruct the patient to take a deep breath and assist exhalation by applying an inferior force to the rib and sidebending the neck toward the side of dysfunction.
4. With the next breath, resist the patient's inhalation by continuing to apply a force to the rib—this holds the rib in exhalation.
5. Again, assist the exhalation by applying even more of a force to the rib and sidebending further.
6. Repeat steps 3 to 5 three to five times.
7. Return the patient to neutral and reassess.

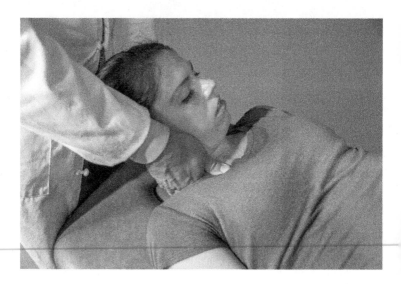

MUSCLE ENERGY—RIBS 3 TO 10 INHALATION DYSFUNCTION

1. The patient lies supine.
2. Stand at the head of the patient and place your thenar and hypothenar eminences at the anterior surface of the ribs (ribs 3 to 5 have more pump handle motion) or lateral surface of the ribs (ribs 6 to 10 have more bucket handle motion).
3. Flex and sidebend the patient toward the side of dysfunction into the barrier.
4. Instruct the patient to take a deep breath.
5. Resist inhalation by applying a counterforce.
6. Assist exhalation by applying a force during the exhalation to bring the patient further into exhalation position with sidebending.
7. Repeat 3 to 5 times.
8. Return the patient to neutral and reassess.

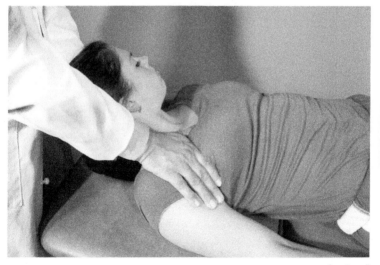

(continued)

Techniques

259

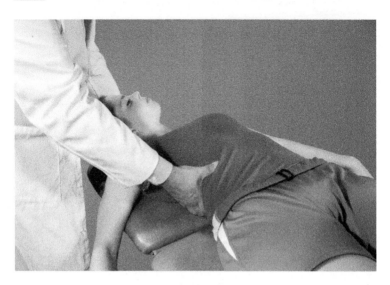

MUSCLE ENERGY USING RESPIRATORY ASSIST— RIBS 11 AND 12 INHALATION DYSFUNCTION

1. The patient lies prone.
2. Stand at the side of the patient, opposite the dysfunction, and place your thenar eminence over the costotransverse articulation of the eleventh and twelfth ribs. Let fingers lie on ribs.
3. Instruct the patient to take a deep breath in and exhale.
4. During exhalation, curl the fingers anteriorly onto the ribs, following the motion of the ribs, to encourage closing of the ribs into normal exhalation position.
5. Repeat steps 3 and 4 three to five times, resisting the ribs motion with inhalation.
6. Reassess.

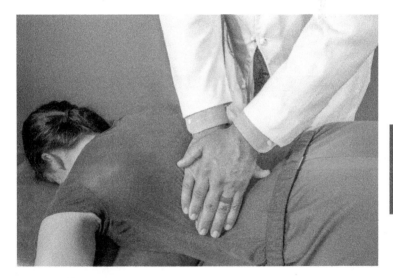

MUSCLE ENERGY—FIRST RIB EXHALATION DYSFUNCTION

1. The patient lies supine.
2. Sit at the head or side of the patient and have the patient place the back of his or her hand on the side of the somatic dysfunction on the patient's forehead.
3. Place one hand over the patient's hand on the head and your other hand beneath the patient to contact rib 1 posteriorly.
4. Ask the patient to inhale and lift his or her head at same time (using anterior and middle scalene muscle).
5. Apply a counterforce to the forehead and apply an inferior force to rib 1 beneath the patient on the posterior aspect of the rib (this will flip the anterior portion of the rib superior and anterior).
6. Repeat steps 4 and 5 three to five times.
7. Return the patient to neutral.
8. Reassess.

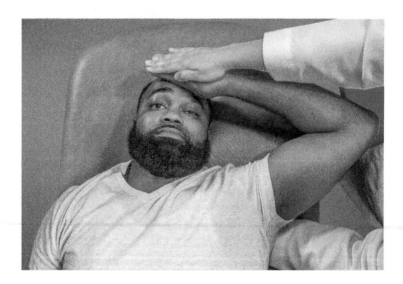

MUSCLE ENERGY—SECOND RIB EXHALATION DYSFUNCTION

1. The patient lies supine.
2. Sit at the head or side of the patient with the patient's head turned away from the dysfunction approximately 30°.
3. Have the patient place the back of his or her hand on the side of the dysfunction on his or her forehead.
4. Place one hand over the patient's hand on the head and your other hand beneath the patient to contact rib 2 posteriorly.
5. Ask the patient to inhale and lift his or her head at same time (using the posterior scalene muscle).
6. Apply a counterforce to the hand on the forehead and an inferior force to posterior aspect of rib 2 beneath the patient.
7. Repeat steps 5 and 6 three to five times.
8. Return the patient to neutral.
9. Reassess.

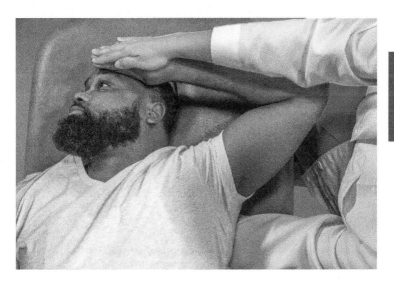

MUSCLE ENERGY—RIBS 3 TO 5 EXHALATION DYSFUNCTION

1. The patient lies supine.
2. Sit at the side of the patient, on the same side as the dysfunction, and have the patient abduct the shoulder and flex the elbow to 90°.
3. Place one arm over the arm of the patient.
4. Place your other hand beneath the patient and contact the rib causing the dysfunction. (Remember! For an exhalation dysfunction, the key rib is the top rib in a group.)
5. Instruct the patient to take a deep breath and lift his or her elbow toward the ceiling at the same time (using the pectoralis muscle minor).
6. Resist this motion with the arm that is lying over the patient's arm and apply inferior traction on the angle of the key rib with the hand on the angle of the rib from beneath the patient, encouraging inhalation motion of the affected ribs.
7. Repeat 3 to 5 times.
8. Reassess.

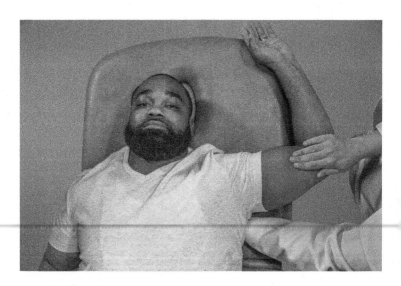

MUSCLE ENERGY—RIBS 6 TO 10 EXHALATION DYSFUNCTION

1. The patient lies supine.
2. Sit at the side of the patient on the same side as the dysfunction.
3. Instruct the patient to abduct the arm on the side of dysfunction and place it at the side of his or her head.
4. Place one hand under the patient at the level of the affected rib and place your other hand (the more cephalad hand) at the patient's elbow.
5. Instruct the patient to take a deep breath.
6. During inhalation, instruct the patient to pull the arm down and across his or her body into your hand (using the serratus anterior muscle).
7. Resist this motion by applying a counterforce and apply inferior traction to the key rib with the hand that is beneath the patient at the angle of the key rib. (This hand encourages inhalation.)
8. Repeat 3 times.
9. Reassess.

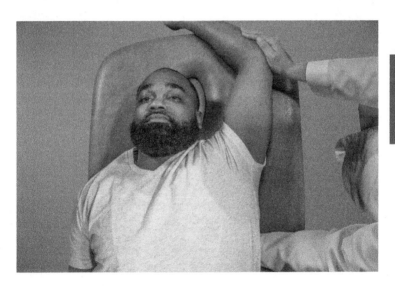

MUSCLE ENERGY—RIBS 11 TO 12 EXHALATION DYSFUNCTION

1. The patient lies prone.
2. Stand at the side of the patient, on the side opposite to the dysfunction, and place your thenar eminence over the eleventh and twelfth ribs.
3. Instruct the patient to inhale deeply (using the quadratus lumborum muscle and the diaphragm).
4. During inhalation, press your thenar eminence anteriorly down into the ribs and then out laterally. Follow the motion of the ribs to encourage opening of the ribs (caliper motion).
5. Repeat steps 3 and 4 three to five times.
6. Reassess.

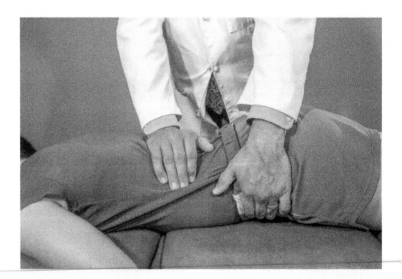

MYOFASCIAL RELEASE/LYMPHATIC—DOMING OF THE DIAPHRAGM

1. The patient lies supine.
2. Standing at the side of the patient, grasp the lower aspects of the patient's rib cage with your palms. Keep your fingers spread apart and your thumb and thenar eminences just below the costal margins. You may use your thumbs to project a vector superiorly up the parasternal costal attachments but do not press on xiphoid process.
3. Have the patient take a deep breath and then exhale.
4. With your thumb and thenar eminences, follow the patient's respiration to gently exaggerate the motion of the diaphragm as well as the rotation and sidebending of the rib cage.
5. Repeat 3 to 5 times; encourage progressively deeper breaths.
6. Reassess.

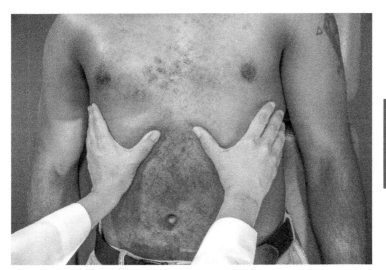

Techniques

MYOFASCIAL RELEASE DIRECT INHIBITION— COLLATERAL GANGLION RELEASE

1. The patient lies supine.

2. Standing at the side of the patient, palpate the regions over the collateral ganglion to be treated (celiac ganglion, figure 1; superior mesenteric, figure 2; inferior mesenteric, figure 3) and evaluate for tissue texture restriction.

3. Assess motion in three plans; move into restriction (barrier).

4. Apply a posterior pressure slowly through the area of tension until a release is felt (or to the limit of patient tolerance).

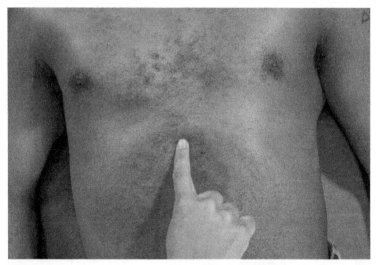

Figure 1

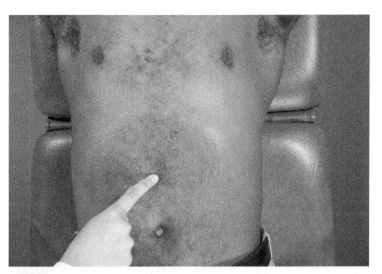

Figure 2

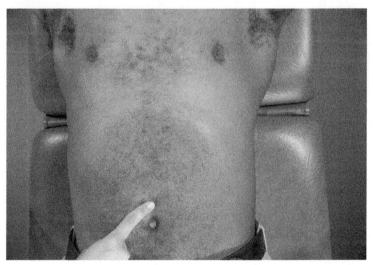

Figure 3

Techniques

DIRECT INHIBITION—CHAPMAN'S REFLEX

1. The patient may be seated or lie supine/prone depending on the location of the reflex point being treated.
2. Standing at the side of the patient, palpate the Chapman point to be treated.
3. Using one finger, apply pressure slowly through the area of tension and tissue texture with a circular motion until a release is felt (or to the limit of patient tolerance).

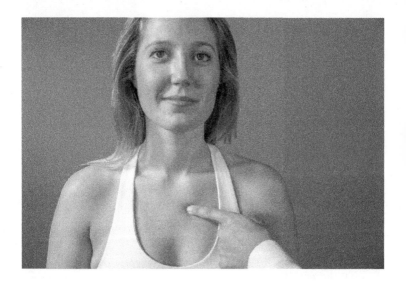

MYOFASCIAL RELEASE—COLONIC STIMULATION

1. The patient lies supine.

2. Standing or sitting at the side of the patient, palpate the length of the colon starting at the sigmoid and working backward toward the cecum.

3. When an area of tissue texture change is palpated, perform the following treatment to the area of somatic dysfunction.

4. Assess motion in three plans; move into restriction (barrier) for a direct technique and away from the restriction (barrier) for an indirect technique.

5. Apply a posterior pressure slowly through the area of tension until a release is felt (or to the limit of patient tolerance). This may take approximately 20 to 60 seconds.

6. Continue to the next area of restriction and repeat steps 4 and 5 until you reach the right lower quadrant near the cecum.

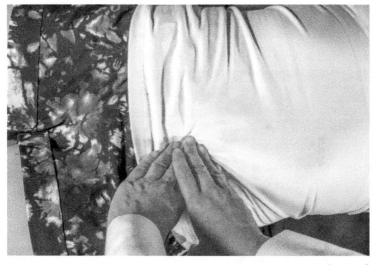

(continued)

Techniques

271

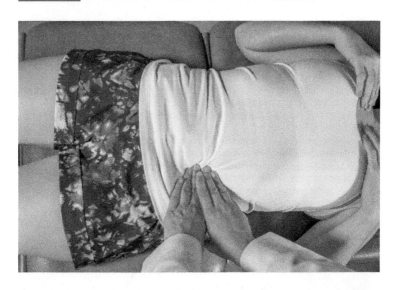

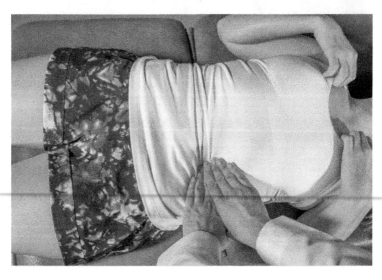

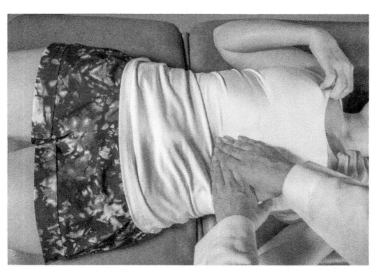

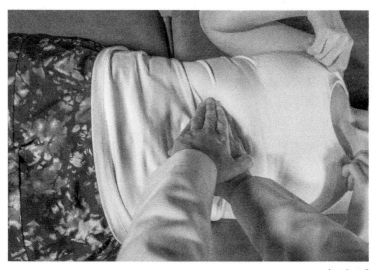

(continued)

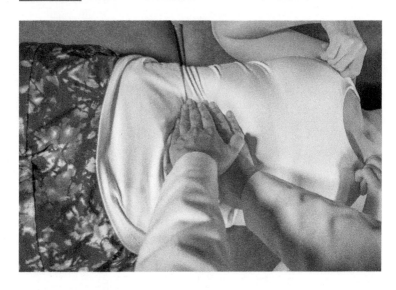

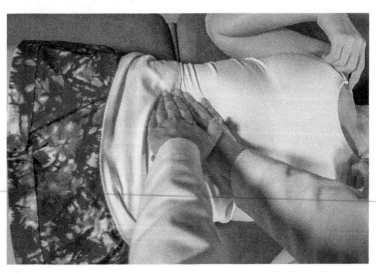

MYOFASCIAL RELEASE DIRECT—MESENTERIC RELEASE/LIFT

1. The patient lies supine.

2. Stand or sit at the right side of the patient

3. Line your fingertips of both hands in a row from the patient's umbilicus to his or her right lower quadrant.

4. Apply a posterior pressure slowly through the area of tension and then gently traction to the patient's right upper quadrant.

5. Hold this tension until a release is felt (or to the limit of patient tolerance). This may take approximately 20 to 60 seconds.

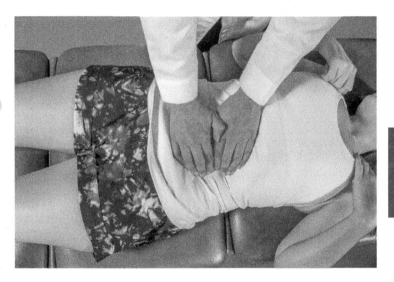

Techniques

Specialized Tests: Head, Cervical, Lumbar, Lower Extremity, Innominate, Sacrum and Upper Extremity

CRANIAL NERVE TESTING

Patient is seated. Sit facing the patient.

CN I: olfactory
Usually not tested but can be evaluated in head trauma when lesions of the anterior fossa (e.g., meningioma) are suspected or when patient reports abnormal smell or taste

- Ask the patient to identify odors (soap, coffee, etc.) at each nostril while the other nostril is occluded.

CN II: optic
Evaluated for clarity of vision, visual fields, optic nerve, and vessel status

- Visual acuity: Test each eye separately on eye chart/card using an eye cover to isolate each eye (if patient wears glasses, do testing with glasses on).
- Visual fields: Examine visual fields by confrontation. Test each eye separately.
  Testing the right eye
  ➤ Face patient, roughly 1 to 2 feet in front of them.
  ➤ Close your right eye while patient closes his or her left.
  ➤ Keep other eyes open and look directly at one another.
  ➤ Move your left arm out (laterally), keeping it equidistant from both of you. A raised index finger should be just outside your field of vision.
  ➤ Wiggle your finger and bring it toward the midline (your noses).
  ➤ You and the patient should see the finger at the same time.
  Testing the left eye
  ➤ Face patient, roughly 1 to 2 feet in front of them.
  ➤ Close your left eye while patient closes his or her right.
  ➤ Keep other eyes open and look directly at one another.
  ➤ Move your right arm out (laterally), keeping it equidistant from both of you. A raised index finger should be just outside your field of vision.
  ➤ Wiggle your finger and bring it toward the midline (your noses).
  ➤ You and the patient should see the finger at the same time.
- Perform funduscopic exam: For each eye, using an ophthalmoscope, evaluate.
  ➤ Optic nerve: for edema (loss of optic nerve borers), cup-to-disc ratio, pallor
  ➤ Macula: edema or exudates
  ➤ Vessels: contour and size, hemorrhage

CN III: oculomotor (pupils, superior rectus, inferior rectus, medial rectus, levator, palpebrae superioris and inferior oblique)
Evaluated for downward and lateral gaze of affected eye. Ask patient if he or she is experiencing diplopia and extraocular movements controlled by these nerves are tested by asking the patient to follow a moving examiner's finger.

- Hold up one index finger in front of the patient's face.
- Test the six cardinal points by making an H pattern in front of the patient.
- Look at pupils: shape, relative size.
- Evaluate eyelid for ptosis.
- Shine light in from the side to gauge pupil's light reaction. Assess both direct and consensual responses.

CN IV: trochlear (superior oblique)
CN V: trigeminal
The three sensory divisions (V1 ophthalmic, V2 maxillary, V3 mandibular) are evaluated by using a pinprick to test facial sensation.

- Corneal reflex: Patient looks up and away.
  - ➤ Lightly touch cotton swab to other side.
  - ➤ Look for blink in both eyes, ask the patient if he or she can sense it.
  - ➤ Repeat other side (tests V sensory, VII motor).
- Facial sensation: sterile sharp item on forehead, cheek, jaw
  - ➤ Repeat with dull object. Ask the patient to report sharp or dull.
- Motor: Patient opens mouth, clenches teeth (pterygoids).
  - ➤ Palpate temporal, masseter muscles as he or she clench.

CN VI: abducens (lateral rectus)
Extraocular movements controlled by these nerves are tested by asking the patient to follow a moving examiner's finger.

- Hold up one index finger in front of the patient's face.
- Test the six cardinal points by making an H pattern in front of the patient.
- Have the patient follow your finger with his or her eyes without moving the head.
- Look for failure of movement, nystagmus.

CN VII: facial
Is evaluated for hemifacial weakness. If the patient has only lower facial weakness (i.e., furrowing of the forehead and eye closure are preserved), etiology of 7th nerve weakness is central rather than peripheral.

- Inspect facial droop or asymmetry.
- Facial expression muscles: Patient looks up and wrinkles forehead.
  - ➤ Examine wrinkling loss.
  - ➤ Feel muscle strength by pushing down on each side (Upper Motor Neuron Lesion preserved because of bilateral innervation).
- Patient shuts eyes tightly: Compare each side.
- Patient grins, frowns, shows teeth, puffs out cheeks: Compare nasolabial grooves.

CN VIII: vestibulocochlear
Hearing loss should prompt formal audiologic testing to confirm findings and distinguish conductive versus sensorineural hearing loss.

- Hearing
  - ➤ Ask the patient if he or she has noticed any difficulty hearing in normal environments.
  - ➤ Hold your hand 1 foot away from the patient's ear.
  - ➤ Rub your fingers together and confirm that the patient can hear the sound.
  - ➤ Repeat on the opposite side.
  - ➤ If indicated, look at external auditory canals, eardrums.
- Vestibular: can be evaluated by testing for nystagmus

CN IX, X: glossopharyngeal, vagus
Usually evaluated together

- Evaluate if the patient's voice is hoarse without apparent infection or post nasal drip.
- Have the patient say "Ahh."
- Look for symmetric palate elevation and uvular displacement (unilateral lesion: palate is paretic on one side and uvula drawn to normal side).
- Gag reflex (sensory [CN IX], motor [CN X]): Stimulate back of throat each side; normal to gag each time

CN XI: accessory
Evaluated by testing the muscles it supplies: SCM and trapezius

- From behind, examine for trapezius atrophy, asymmetry.
- Patient shrugs shoulders (trapezius).
- Patient turns head against resistance (SCM).

CN XII: hypoglossal
Evaluated by testing the muscles it supplies: glossal muscle (tongue)

- Listen for clarity of patient's speech.
- Inspect tongue in mouth for wasting, fasciculations.
- Protrude tongue: unilateral deviates to affected side.

Specialized Tests

TEMPOROMANDIBULAR JOINT EVALUATION

Evaluation of TMJ motion should be performed on all patients with headaches and neck pain. Joint arthritis, deformities of the mandibular condyles, and pterygoid hypertonicity can cause deviation/dysfunction.

- The patient is seated.
- While facing the patient, ask the patient to slowly open his or her jaw as wide as he or she can and to slowly close it.[1]
- Watch for deviations of the mandible from the midline during opening and closing.

Negative test: Mandible stays in the midline during opening and closing.
Positive test: Mandible deviates from the midline, swinging to one side or in a zigzag pattern as the patient opens and closes his or her jaw.

---

[1]*Dysfunctions will be missed if the patient opens and closes too quickly or if he or she does not open his or her jaws fully.*

DISTRACTION TEST

Is a diagnostic test for the presence of cervical radiculopathy. If radicular symptoms are relieved as a result of cephalad traction, then the test is positive for nerve root compression (e.g., herniated disc or facet arthropathy).

Negative test: Pain is unchanged with traction.
Positive test: Pain is relieved with traction, indicating nerve root compression.

1. The patient is seated.
2. Stand at the side of the patient, cup the patient's chin and occiput with your hands, and pull cephalward.
3. The test result is positive if pain is relieved.

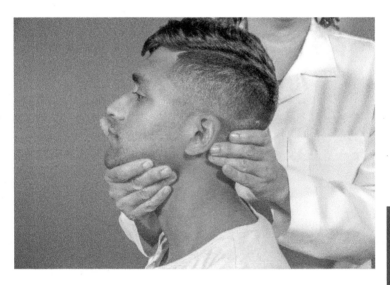

POTENTIAL SOMATIC DYSFUNCTIONS ASSOCIATED WITH THIS TEST

Radicular pain symptoms may also be caused by hypertonicity of the paraspinal musculature of the cervical and thoracic spine.

CERVICAL COMPRESSION TEST (SPURLING'S TEST)

Is a provocative test for the presence of cervical radiculopathy. If radicular symptoms are produced as a result of caudad axial compression, then the test is positive for nerve root compression (e.g., herniated disc or facet arthropathy).

Negative test: No radicular symptoms with compression
Positive test: Pain is caused with axial compression.

1. The patient is seated.
2. Stand behind the patient.
3. Clasp your fingers and gently press down on the top of the patient's head.
4. The test result is positive if radicular pain is elicited.

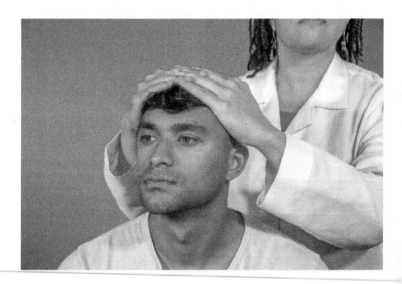

VALSALVA TEST

Is a provocative test for the presence of cervical radiculopathy. The maneuver increases intrathecal pressure. If radicular symptoms are produced as a result of the maneuver, then the test is positive for nerve root compression (e.g., herniated disc, spinal cord tumor, any space-occupying lesion).

Negative test: No radicular symptoms with maneuver
Positive test: Pain is caused by maneuver.

1. The patient is seated.
2. Instruct the patient to take a deep breath and bear down.
3. The test result is positive if pain is elicited.

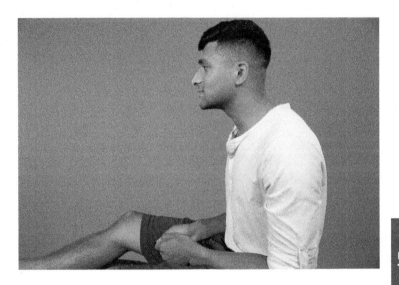

SWALLOWING TEST (POSSIBLE INFECTION, OSTEOPHYTES, HEMATOMA, OR TUMOR IN THE ANTERIOR PORTION OF THE CERVICAL SPINE)

Negative test: No pain or difficulty swallowing
Positive test: The test result is positive if the patient has pain or difficulty swallowing.[2]

1. The patient is seated.
2. Instruct the patient to swallow.

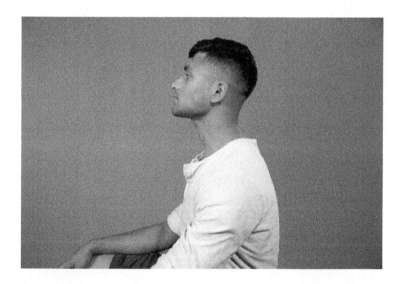

[2]Assumes no other clear causes of such as pharyngitis, etc.

TRENDELENBURG'S TEST (GLUTEUS MEDIUS WEAKNESS)

1. The patient is standing, facing away from the physician.
2. Instruct the patient to raise one leg off the floor.

Negative test: The test is negative for gluteus medius weakness on the weight-bearing leg if the hips stay level.
Positive test: The test is positive for gluteus medius weakness on the weight-bearing leg if the hip drops down on the side of the raised leg.

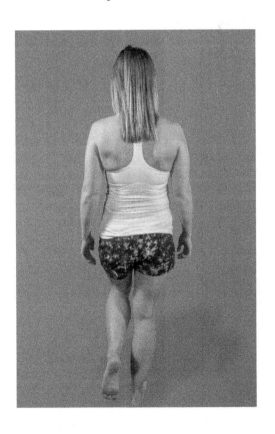

KNEE EXAM—ANTERIOR DRAWER TEST
(ANTERIOR CRUCIATE LIGAMENT TEAR)

1. The patient lies supine.
2. Instruct the patient to flex hips to 45°, bend knees to 90°, and keep feet flat on the table.
3. Sit on the side of knee being evaluated and stabilize the foot by sitting at its edge.
4. Wrap both hands around the tibia with one thumb on the medial joint line and one on the lateral joint line.
5. Pull the tibia anteriorly.

Negative test: The joint feels stable without laxity.
Positive test: The test result is positive if there is laxity and the tibia comes out from under the femur.

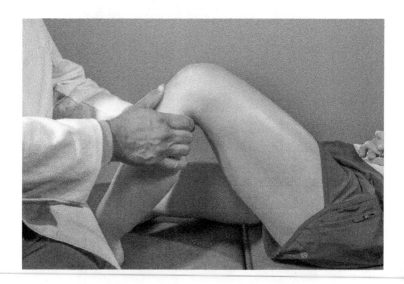

KNEE EXAM—POSTERIOR DRAWER TEST
(POSTERIOR CRUCIATE LIGAMENT TEAR)

1. The patient lies supine.

2. Instruct the patient to flex hips to 45°, bend knees to 90°, and keep feet flat on the table.

3. Sit on the side of knee being evaluated and stabilize the foot by sitting at its edge.

4. Wrap both hands around the tibia with one thumb on the medial joint line and one on the lateral joint line.

5. Push the tibia posteriorly.

Negative test: The joint feels stable without laxity.
Positive test: The test result is positive if there is laxity and the tibia goes backward under the femur.

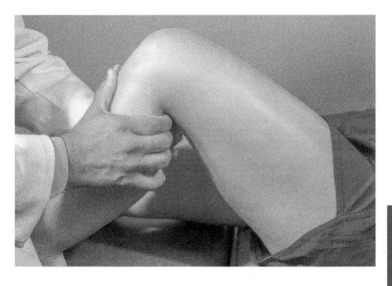

APLEY'S COMPRESSION TEST (MENISCAL TEARS)

1. The patient lies prone.
2. Instruct the patient to flex the knee to 90°.
3. Press down on the patient's heel while internally and externally rotating the leg.

Negative test: No pain elicited
Positive test: The test result is positive for a meniscal tear if this elicits pain.

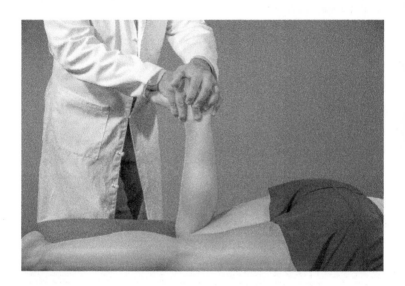

APLEY'S DISTRACTION TEST (LIGAMENTOUS TEARS)

1. The patient lies prone.
2. Instruct the patient to flex the knee to 90°.
3. Hold the distal femur down with one hand.
4. With the other hand, pull up on the patient's heel while internally and externally rotating the leg.

Negative test: No pain elicited
Positive test: The test result is positive for a ligamentous tear if this elicits pain.

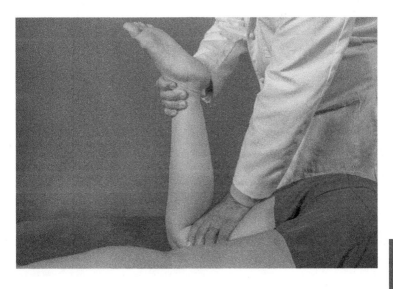

LACHMAN'S TEST
(ANTERIOR CRUCIATE LIGAMENT TEAR)

1. The patient lies supine.
2. Grasp the patient's proximal tibia with one hand and stabilize the distal femur with the other hand.
3. Pull the tibia anteriorly.

Negative test: The joint feels stable without laxity.
Positive test: The test result is positive if there is laxity and the tibia comes out from under the femur.

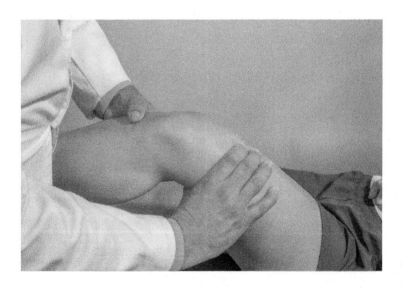

McMURRAY'S TEST
(POSTERIOR TEAR OF THE MEDIAL MENISCUS)

1. The patient lies supine.
2. Instruct the patient to flex the knee to 90°.
3. Grasp the patient's heel with one hand and the knee with the other.
4. Externally rotate the tibia while applying a valgus stress to the knee.
5. Slowly extend the knee.

Negative test: No pain elicited
Positive test: The test result is positive if there is an audible click or the patient feels pain.

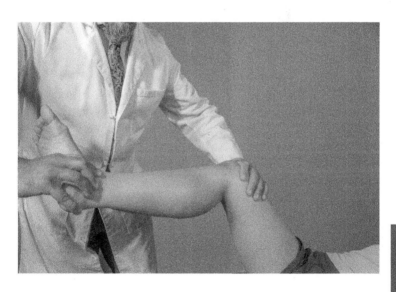

Specialized Tests

McMURRAY'S TEST (TEAR OF THE LATERAL MENISCUS)

1. The patient lies supine.
2. Instruct the patient to flex the knee to 90°.
3. Grasp the patient's heel with one hand and the knee with the other.
4. Internally rotate the tibia while applying a varus stress to the knee.
5. Slowly extend the knee.

Negative test: No pain elicited
Positive test: The test result is positive if there is an audible click or the patient feels pain.

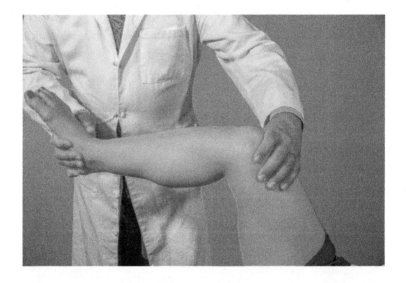

PATELLAR GRIND TEST (CHONDROMALACIA)

1. The patient lies supine.
2. Push the patella inferiorly and hold it there.
3. Instruct the patient to contract his or her quadriceps muscles.

Negative test: No pain or palpable grind
Positive test: The test result is positive if the patient feels pain or there is palpable grind.

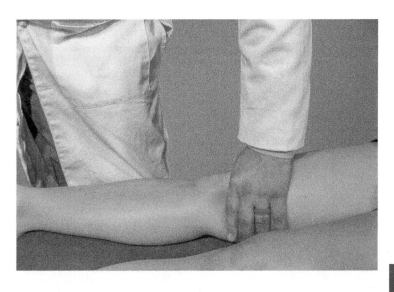

Specialized Tests

VALGUS STRESS
(MEDIAL COLLATERAL LIGAMENT TEAR)

1. The patient lies supine.
2. Instruct the patient to slightly flex the knee.
3. Hold the patient's ankle with one hand and place your hand on the lateral knee.
4. Apply a medial (valgus) stress.

Negative test: The joint feels stable without laxity.
Positive test: The test result is positive if there is medial gapping of the joint.

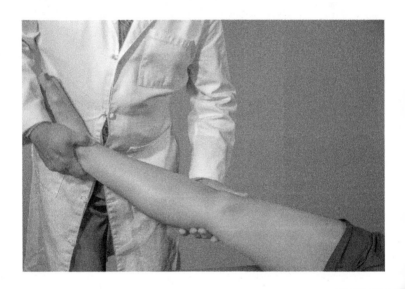

VARUS STRESS
(LATERAL COLLATERAL LIGAMENT TEAR)

1. The patient lies supine.
2. Instruct the patient to slightly flex the knee.
3. Hold the patient's ankle with one hand and place your hand on the medial knee.
4. Apply a lateral (varus) stress.

Negative test: The joint feels stable without laxity.
Positive test: The test result is positive if there is lateral gapping of the joint.

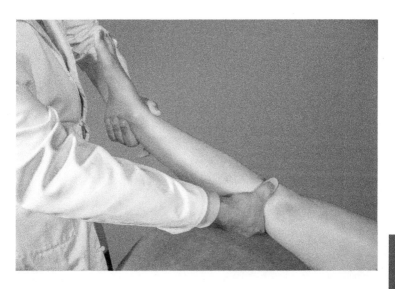

ANTERIOR DRAWER TEST FOR ANKLE INSTABILITY (TEAR OF ANTERIOR TALOFIBULAR LIGAMENT AND POSSIBLY OTHER LIGAMENTS)

1. The patient lies supine.
2. Cup the posterior calcaneus and grasp the tibia and fibula with either hand.
3. Attempt to draw the foot anterior in relation to the mortise joint.
4. Compare to uninjured ankle.

Negative test: The joint feels stable without laxity.
Positive test: The test result is positive if there is laxity and the foot is drawn anterior in relation to the mortise joint.

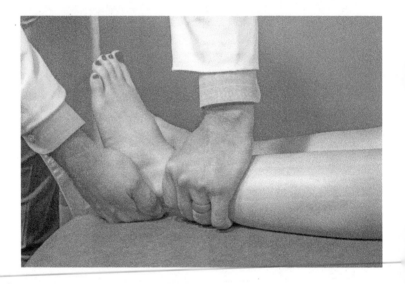

POTENTIAL SOMATIC DYSFUNCTIONS ASSOCIATED WITH THIS TEST

An anterior tibia on a talus somatic dysfunction of the lower extremity may appear to be a slightly positive anterior drawer test at the ankle.

STRAIGHT LEG RAISING TEST

Evaluation of radicular symptoms caused by compression of the sciatic nerve due to lumbar disk herniation

Normal (negative test) with elevation of the leg up to 70° and dorsiflexion of the foot, there is no reproduction of pain into the lower leg

1. The patient lies supine.
2. Stand at the side of the patient, grasp the heel of the side being tested, and place the other hand over the knee (keeping the knee extended).
3. Flex the leg at the hip to approximately 70° or until the patient feels discomfort.
4. If less than 70° of hip flexion is achieved, lower the leg to just below the level where pain was elicited.
5. Dorsiflex the foot.
6. The test result is positive if dorsiflexion of the foot at less than 70° elicits pain all the way down the leg in a radicular pattern.

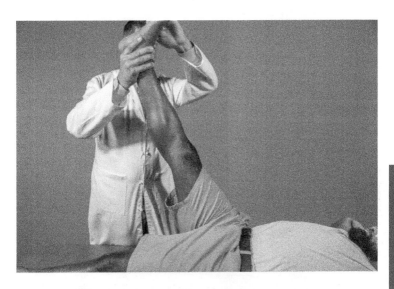

POTENTIAL SOMATIC DYSFUNCTIONS ASSOCIATED WITH THIS TEST

Muscles running adjacent to or around the sciatic nerve that are hypertonic may compress or irritate the nerve.

1. Piriformis
2. Hamstring muscles
   a. Semitendinosus
   b. Semimembranosus
   c. Biceps femoris

Specialized Tests

HIP DROP TEST

Evaluation of the lumbar spine's ability to sidebend
     Normal (negative test) results in the iliac crest dropping greater than 25° (indicates the lumbar spine sidebending away from the bent knee)
     Abnormal (positive test) iliac crest drops less than 20° (indicates the lumbar spine sidebending toward the bent knee).

1. The patient is standing.
2. Locate the lateral aspect of the iliac crest.
3. Instruct the patient to bend one knee without lifting his or her heel off the floor.
4. The test result is positive for sidebending toward the bended knee if the patient's ipsilateral hip drops less than 25°.

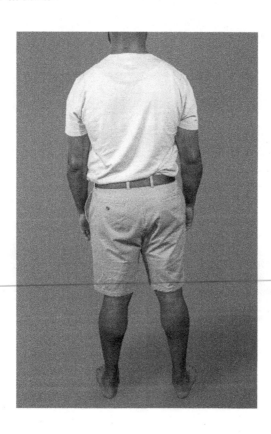

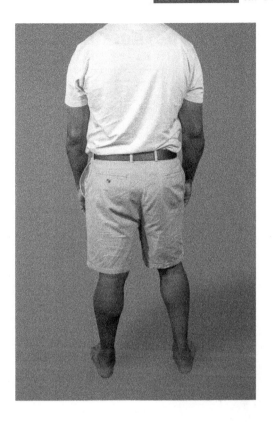

POTENTIAL SOMATIC DYSFUNCTIONS ASSOCIATED WITH THIS TEST

Somatic dysfunction of the lumbars is the primary cause of a positive test result. Hypertonicity of musculature may be the underlying cause of sidebending in the lumbar spine to the side that drops the least.

Muscles that may be involved include:

1. Psoas.
2. Quadratus lumborum.
3. Paraspinal postural muscles.

Specialized Tests

ASIS COMPRESSION TEST (LOCATES THE SIDE OF SOMATIC DYSFUNCTION IN THE PELVIS)

1. The patient lies supine.
2. Stand next to the patient with the dominant eye over the midline.
3. Place your palms over each ASIS.
4. Apply a posterior compression to each ASIS one at a time, feeling for the quantity and quality of motion in each side.
5. The test result is positive for dysfunction on the side that is least mobile or feels restricted to the motion testing.

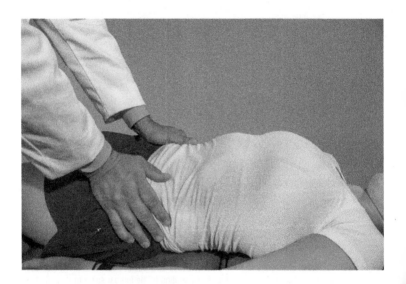

POTENTIAL SOMATIC DYSFUNCTIONS ASSOCIATED WITH THIS TEST

This is a lateralizing test for sacroiliac joint dysfunction. A positive test result may be indicative of an innominate or a sacral dysfunction. Innominate and sacral landmarks will further diagnose the somatic dysfunction.

STANDING FLEXION TEST (LOCATES THE SIDE OF SOMATIC DYSFUNCTION IN THE PELVIS)

1. The patient is standing.
2. Locate the patient's PSISs.
3. Sit or bend so that your eyes are at the level of the PSISs.
4. Place each thumb under the inferior notch of the PSISs.
5. Instruct the patient to bend forward slowly (without bending the knees).
6. The test result is positive if one PSIS moves more superiorly than the other at the end of forward bending.

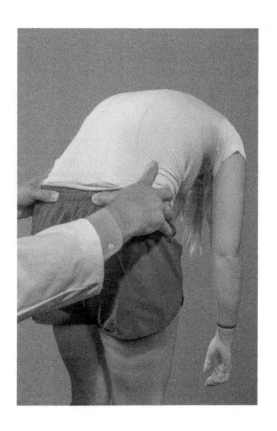

POTENTIAL SOMATIC DYSFUNCTIONS ASSOCIATED WITH THIS TEST

Innominate dysfunctions are most likely to cause a positive standing flexion test result; however, a sacral dysfunction, a pubic dysfunction, or tight hamstrings on the contralateral side may cause a positive test result.

SEATED FLEXION TEST (LOCATES THE SIDE OF SOMATIC DYSFUNCTION IN THE PELVIS, ESPECIALLY THE SACRUM)

1. The patient is seated.
2. Locate the patient's PSISs.
3. Place each thumb under the inferior notch of the PSISs.
4. Sitting behind the patient with your eyes at the level of the PSISs is helpful.
5. Instruct the patient to bend forward slowly.
6. The test result is positive if one PSIS moves more superiorly than the other at the end of forward bending.

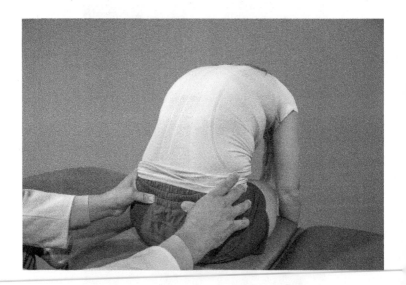

POTENTIAL SOMATIC DYSFUNCTIONS ASSOCIATED WITH THIS TEST

Sacral dysfunction will cause a positive test result. It determines the side of the dysfunctional sacroiliac joint. In the case of a torsion, the positive side is opposite of the involved oblique axis.

LUMBOSACRAL SPRING TEST (POSTERIOR SACRAL BASE)

1. The patient lies prone and then props himself or herself up on his or her elbows.
2. Place the heel of the hand at the base of the lumbosacral junction.
3. The test result is positive if there is little or no springing.

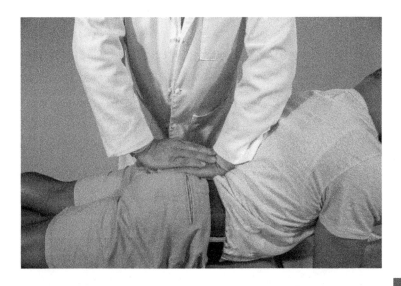

POTENTIAL SOMATIC DYSFUNCTIONS ASSOCIATED WITH THIS TEST

A positive spring test result indicates a flexed L5 and an extended sacral base. This occurs in either a posterior torsion (left on right, right on left) or unilateral or bilateral sacral extension dysfunction.

Specialized Tests

APLEY'S SCRATCH TEST (SHOULDER RANGE OF MOTION)

1. The patient is seated.
2. Instruct the patient to reach behind his or her head and touch the opposite scapula (abduction/external rotation).
3. Instruct the patient to then reach behind his or her back and touch the inferior angle of the opposite scapula (internal rotation/adduction).
4. Repeat with other shoulder and compare for asymmetry and significant loss of motion.

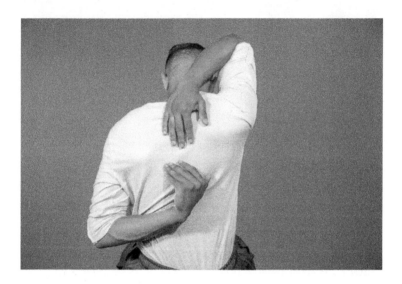

POTENTIAL SOMATIC DYSFUNCTIONS ASSOCIATED WITH THIS TEST

Hypertonicity of rotator cuff muscles and other muscles of the shoulder can lead to decreased motion. A hypertonic muscle will exaggerate its normal motion and restrict the antagonistic motion.

Muscle	Normal Function/Somatic Dysfunction Caused by Hypertonicity	Restriction Caused by Hypertonicity
Supraspinatus	Abduction	Adduction
Infraspinatus	External rotation	Internal rotation
Teres minor	External rotation	Internal rotation
Subscapularis	Internal rotation/extension	External rotation/flexion
Teres major	Internal rotation/adduction	External rotation/abduction
Deltoid	Abduction, flexion and extension	Adduction, flexion and extension

DROP ARM TEST (ROTATOR CUFF TEARS, ESPECIALLY SUPRASPINATUS)

1. The patient is seated.
2. Instruct the patient to abduct his or her arm to 90° and then slowly lower the arm to his or her side.
3. The test result is positive if the patient cannot lower the arm smoothly or if the arm drops to the side.

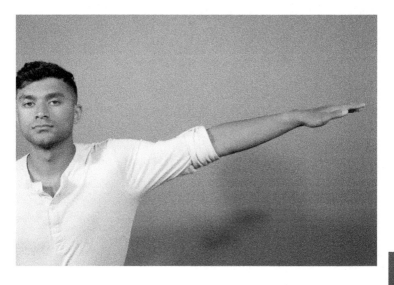

NEER'S TEST (IMPINGEMENT OF SUPRASPINATUS AND INFRASPINATUS TENDONS UNDER ACROMION PROCESS)

1. The patient is seated with shoulder abducted to 90° from the body.
2. Physician passively continues to abduct shoulder.
3. A positive test elicits pain under acromion process.

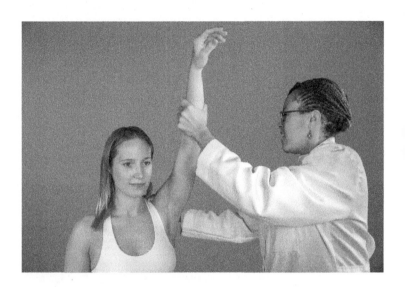

HAWKIN'S TEST (IMPINGEMENT OF SUPRASPINATUS AND INFRASPINATUS TENDONS UNDER ACROMION PROCESS)

1. The patient is seated with elbow flexed to 90° and shoulder abducted to 90°.
2. Physician passively abducts and internally rotates the shoulder.
3. A positive test elicits pain under acromion process.

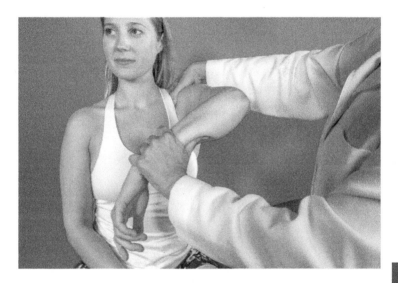

SPEED'S TEST (BICEPS TENDONITIS, ENTHESOPATHY, OR LABRAL TEAR)

1. Patient is seated with elbow extended, forearm supinated, and shoulder flexed to 90°.
2. Physician controls the elbow and wrist and asks the patient to attempt to flex elbow by contracting biceps muscle.
3. A positive test elicits pain in the biceps or shoulder.

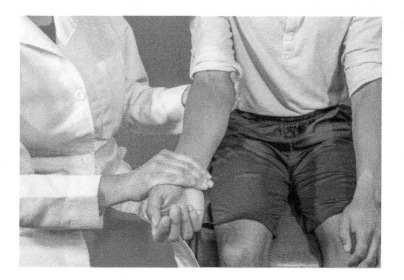

YERGASON'S TEST (STABILITY OF THE BICEPS TENDON IN THE BICIPITAL GROOVE)

1. The patient is seated.
2. Stand behind the patient and instruct the patient to flex his or her elbow to 90°.
3. Grasp the patient's arm at the elbow with one hand and at the wrist with your other hand.
4. Pull inferiorly at the patient's elbow while externally rotating the forearm.
5. Instruct the patient to resist the external rotation.
6. The test result is positive if pain is elicited at the biceps tendon as it comes out of the bicipital groove.

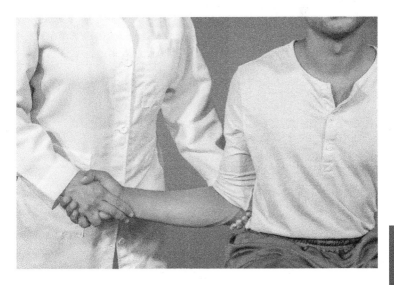

APPREHENSION TEST (ANTERIOR GLENOHUMERAL INSTABILITY)

1. The patient is seated.
2. Stand behind the patient, and with the patient's shoulder at 90° of abduction and elbow flexion, apply slight anterior pressure to the humerus and externally rotate the arm.
3. The test result is positive if this elicits pain or apprehension about the feeling of impending dislocation.

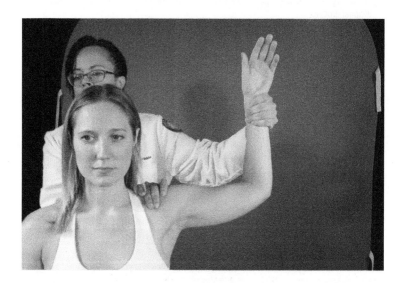

ADSON'S TEST (THORACIC OUTLET SYNDROME) (BRACHIAL PLEXUS IMPINGEMENT BETWEEN ANTERIOR AND MIDDLE SCALENE)

1. The patient is seated.
2. Stand behind the patient and monitor the radial pulse.
3. Slightly abduct the arm and extend it at the shoulder and elbow.
4. Externally rotate the patient's arm.
5. Instruct the patient to look toward the ipsilateral side.
6. The test result is positive if the radial pulse significantly decreases or becomes absent or if the test exacerbates the patient's pain or paresthesia.

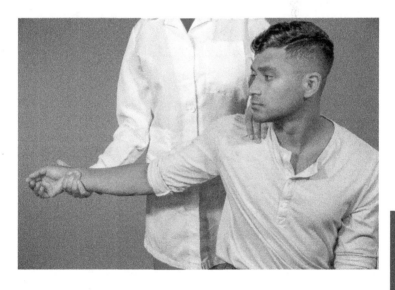

POTENTIAL SOMATIC DYSFUNCTIONS ASSOCIATED WITH THIS TEST

Hypertonic scalene muscles that run adjacent to or around the brachial plexus may compress or irritate the nerve.

- Anterior scalene
- Middle scalene
- Rib 1

Specialized Tests

MILITARY POSTURE TEST (COSTOCLAVICULAR SYNDROME TEST) (BRACHIAL PLEXUS IMPINGEMENT BETWEEN CLAVICLE AND FIRST RIB)

1. The patient is seated.
2. Stand behind the patient and palpate the radial pulse and extend the shoulder with one hand while depressing the clavicle and the shoulder with the other hand.
3. The test result is positive if the radial pulse significantly decreases or is absent or if the test exacerbates the patient's pain or paresthesia.

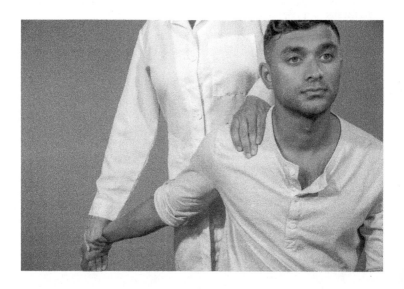

POTENTIAL SOMATIC DYSFUNCTIONS ASSOCIATED WITH THIS TEST

Somatic dysfunction of the clavicle or first rib can irritate the brachial plexus.

WRIGHT'S TEST (BRACHIAL PLEXUS IMPINGEMENT UNDER PECTORALIS MINOR)

1. The patient is seated.
2. Stand behind the patient and palpate the radial pulse with one hand.
3. Abduct the patient's arm above his or her head with external rotation and extension.
4. The test result is positive if the radial pulse significantly decreases or is absent or if the test exacerbates the patient's pain or paresthesia.

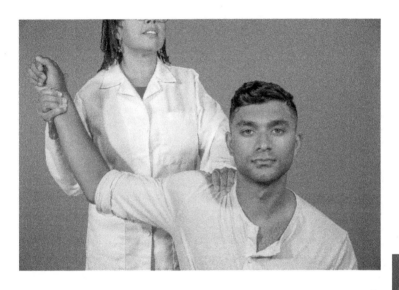

POTENTIAL SOMATIC DYSFUNCTIONS ASSOCIATED WITH THIS TEST

If the pectoralis minor, which runs adjacent to the brachial plexus, is hypertonic, the brachial plexus may be compressed or irritated.

Specialized Tests

TINEL'S SIGN AT ELBOW (ULNAR NERVE ENTRAPMENT)

1. The patient is seated.
2. Tap posterior to the medial epicondyle of the elbow.
3. A positive test result produces painful symptoms in ulnar nerve distribution (fourth and fifth digits).

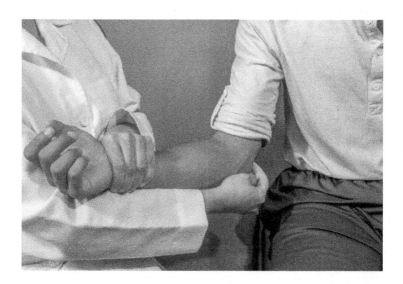

POTENTIAL SOMATIC DYSFUNCTIONS ASSOCIATED WITH THIS TEST

The ulnar nerve may be compromised by the following:

- Hypertonic wrist flexors
- Flexor digitorum
- Dysfunction of the ulna bone

COZEN'S TEST—TENNIS ELBOW TEST (LATERAL EPICONDYLITIS)

1. The patient is seated.
2. The physician faces the patient.
3. With the patient's arm pronated and elbow flexed, instruct the patient to extend his or her wrist. Then have the patient attempt to maintain wrist extension against resistance.
4. Pain at the lateral epicondyle indicates lateral epicondylitis.

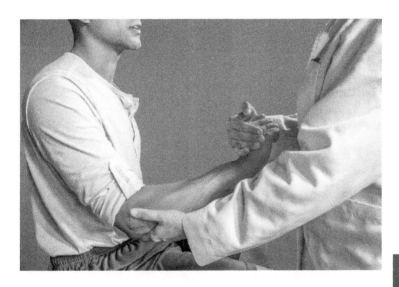

Specialized Tests

MILL'S TEST—TENNIS ELBOW TEST (LATERAL EPICONDYLITIS)

1. The patient is seated.
2. The physician faces the patient.
3. The patient begins with their forearm pronated and elbow flexed to 90 degrees.
4. The physician palpates the lateral epicondyle and passively flexes the wrist and pronates the patient's forearm.
5. A positive test is reproduction of pain at the lateral epicondyle.

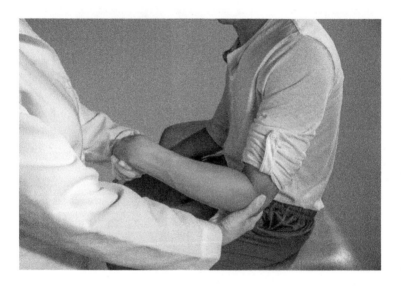

POTENTIAL SOMATIC DYSFUNCTIONS ASSOCIATED WITH THIS TEST

The forearm extensor muscles attach at the lateral epicondyle. Hypertonicity and tenderpoints of the forearm extensor muscles may be associated with lateral epicondylitis.

GOLFER'S ELBOW TEST (MEDIAL EPICONDYLITIS)

1. The patient is seated.
2. The physician faces the patient.
3. With the elbow flexed and the forearm supinated, extend the patient's wrist.
4. Use your other hand to palpate the medial epicondyle while you maintain wrist extension and fully extend the patient's elbow.
5. A positive test causes pain at the medial epicondyle.

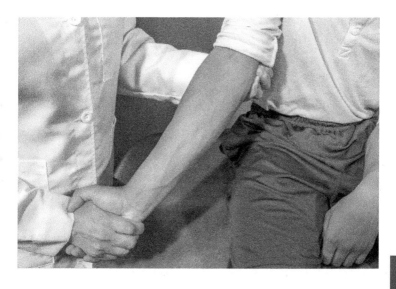

POTENTIAL SOMATIC DYSFUNCTIONS ASSOCIATED WITH THIS TEST

The forearm flexor muscles attach at the medial epicondyle. Hypertonicity and tenderpoints of the forearm extensor muscles may be associated with medial epicondylitis.

Specialized Tests

TESTS FOR LIGAMENTOUS STABILITY AT ELBOW

1. The patient is seated.
2. The physician faces the patient.
3. With the patient's elbow extended, grasp the patient's wrist and distal humerus.
4. Apply first a valgus stress and then a varus stress to the elbow.
5. The test result is positive if there is excessive motion indicating a tear of the collateral ligament (valgus stress = medial collateral ligament; varus stress = lateral collateral ligament).

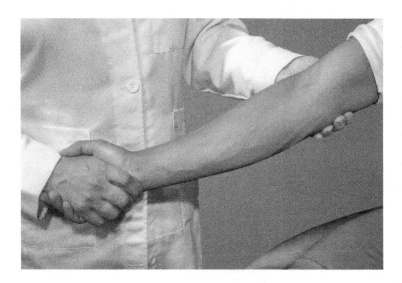

ALLEN'S TEST (ARTERIAL INSUFFICIENCY OF THE RADIAL AND ULNAR ARTERIES TO THE HAND)

1. The patient is seated.
2. Occlude the patient's radial and ulnar arteries at the wrist.
3. Instruct the patient to open and close his or her hand several times and then make a tight fist.
4. Instruct the patient to open his or her hand. (The palm should be pale.)
5. Release one of the arteries. (The patient's hand should flush.)
6. The test result is positive if the hand flushes slowly or not at all.
7. Repeat the above steps for the other artery.

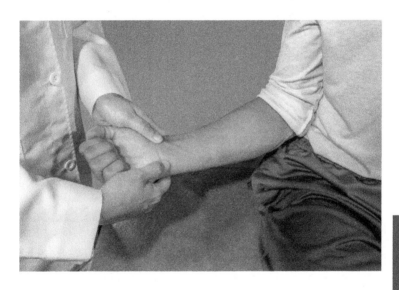

POTENTIAL SOMATIC DYSFUNCTIONS ASSOCIATED WITH THIS TEST

Arterial supply may be compromised by the following:

- Dysfunctional carpal bones
- Hypertonic wrist flexors
- Dysfunction of the radius and ulna bones

Specialized Tests

FINKELSTEIN'S TEST (DE QUERVAIN'S DISEASE/TENOSYNOVITIS)

1. The patient is seated.
2. Instruct the patient to make a fist with the thumb tucked under the fingers.
3. Stabilize the patient's forearm and deviate the wrist toward the ulna.
4. The test result is positive if the patient feels pain over the radial tendons of the wrist.

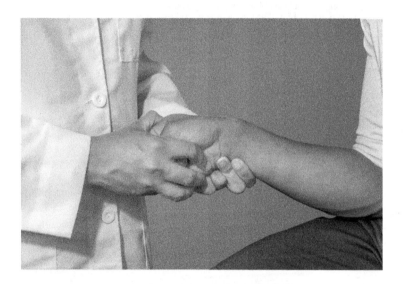

POTENTIAL SOMATIC DYSFUNCTIONS ASSOCIATED WITH THIS TEST

Hypertonic and overused abductor pollicis longus and extensor pollicis brevis can cause irritation of their associated tendons.

PHALEN'S TEST (CARPAL TUNNEL SYNDROME)

1. The patient is seated.
2. The patient flexes his or her wrists as far as possible and holds this position for 1 minute.
3. The test result is positive if paresthesias are felt in the distribution of the median nerve (fingers 1 to 3 and radial aspect of the fourth digit).

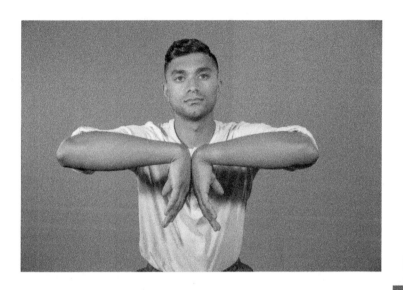

POTENTIAL SOMATIC DYSFUNCTIONS ASSOCIATED WITH THIS TEST

The median nerve may be compromised by the following:

- Dysfunctional carpal bones
- Hypertonic wrist flexors
- Dysfunction of the radius and ulna bones
- Facial strain of flexor retinaculum

Specialized Tests

TINEL'S SIGN AT WRIST (CARPAL TUNNEL SYNDROME)

1. The patient is seated.
2. Extend the patient's wrist and tap on the volar aspect of the wrist.
3. The test result is positive if paresthesias are felt in the distribution of the median nerve (fingers 1 to 3 and radial aspect of the fourth digit).

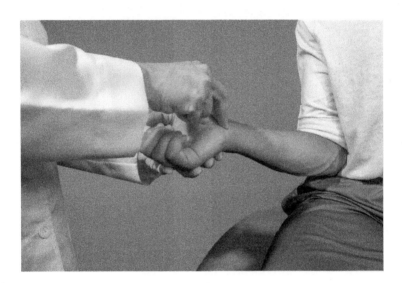

POTENTIAL SOMATIC DYSFUNCTIONS ASSOCIATED WITH THIS TEST

The median nerve may be compromised by the following:

- Dysfunctional carpal bones
- Hypertonic wrist flexors
- Dysfunction of the radius and ulna bones

Summary Charts

POTENTIAL UPPER EXTREMITY NERVE IMPINGEMENTS

1. Upper and lower trunk of the brachial plexus by the scalene muscles
2. Lower trunk of the brachial plexus by an inhalation dysfunction of the first rib or clavicle dysfunction
3. Lower trunk of the brachial plexus by pectoralis minor
4. Median nerve by pronator teres somatic dysfunction
5. Ulnar nerve by wrist flexor somatic dysfunction (associated with medial epicondylitis)
6. Radial nerve by the radial head somatic dysfunction or radial nerve by wrist extensor somatic dysfunction (associated with lateral epicondylitis)
7. Ulnar nerve with somatic dysfunction of the carpal bones
8. Median nerve by somatic dysfunction of the carpal bones and with carpal tunnel syndrome

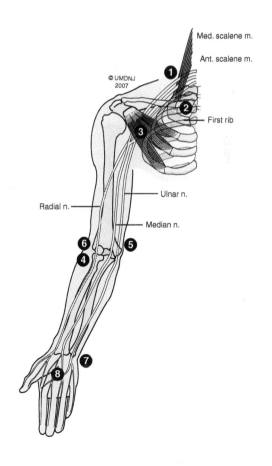

POTENTIAL LOWER EXTREMITY NERVE IMPINGEMENTS

1. Femoral nerve by psoas
2. Sciatic nerve by piriformis or hamstring muscles
3. Common fibular nerve by fibular head somatic dysfunction
4. Deep fibular nerve by somatic dysfunction of the anterior compartment of the leg
5. Iliohypogastric/ilioinguinal, genitofemoral, and/or lateral femoral cutaneous nerve by the iliolumbar ligaments, lumbar or innominate somatic dysfunctions
6. Tibial nerve at the tarsal tunnel

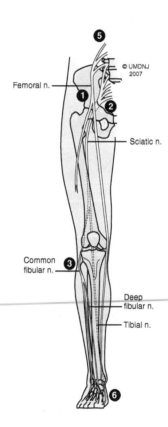

© UMDNJ
2007

Femoral n.

Sciatic n.

Common fibular n.

Deep fibular n.

Tibial n.

ANTERIOR DERMATOMES

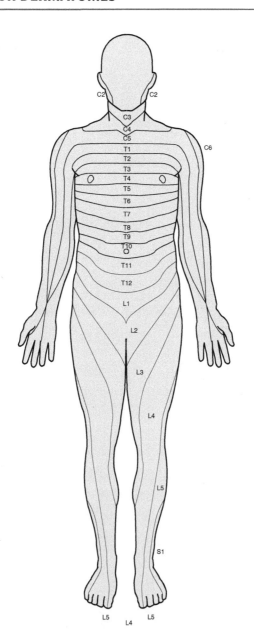

POSTERIOR DERMATOMES

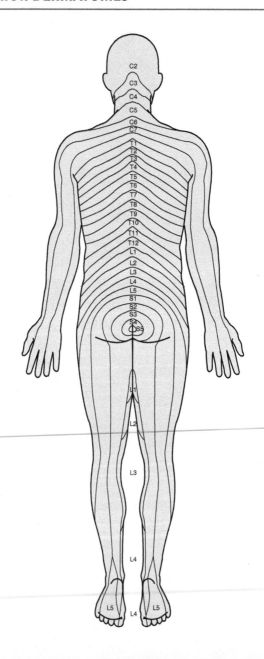

REFLEXES

UPPER EXTREMITY

Reflexes	Nerve Root
Biceps reflex	C5–C6

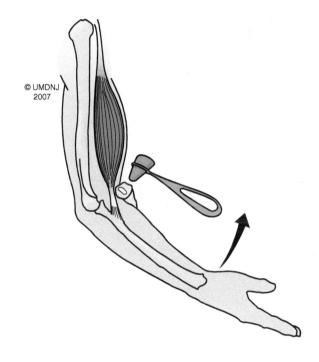

© UMDNJ
2007

Reflexes	Nerve Root
Brachioradialis reflex	C6

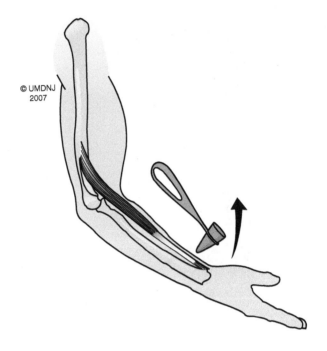

© UMDNJ
2007

Reflexes	Nerve Root
Triceps reflex	C7

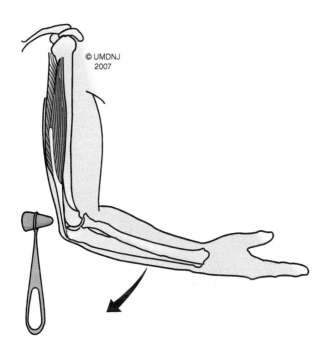

© UMDNJ
2007

REFLEXES

LOWER EXTREMITY

Reflexes	Nerve Root
Patellar reflex	L4

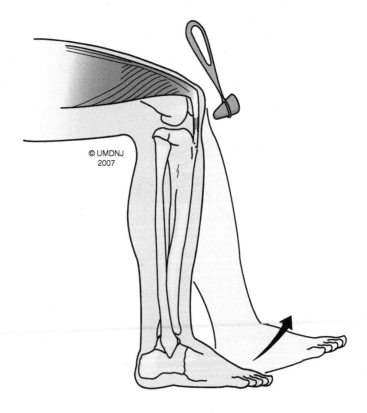

© UMDNJ
2007

Reflexes	Nerve Root
Achilles reflex	S1

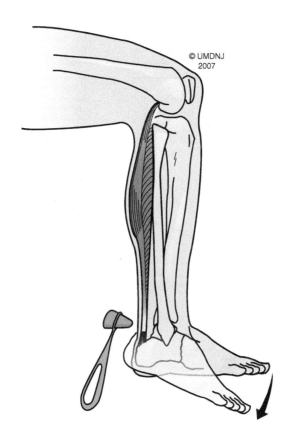

© UMDNJ
2007

MUSCLE STRENGTH

UPPER EXTREMITY

Muscle Motion	Muscle	Nerve	Nerve Root
Arm abduction	Deltoid	Axillary	C5–C6

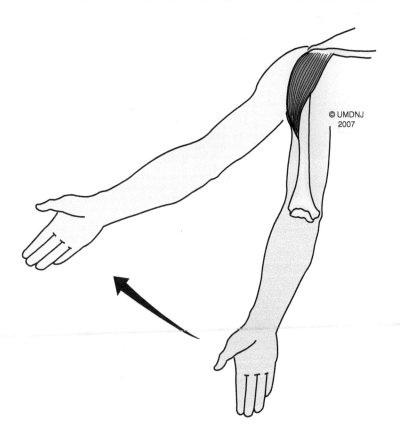

© UMDNJ
2007

Muscle Motion	Muscle	Nerve	Nerve Root
Elbow flexion	Biceps	Musculocutaneous	C5–C6

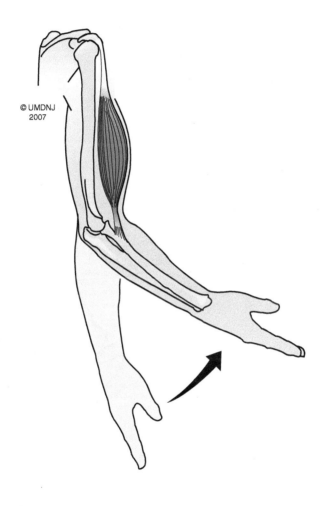

© UMDNJ
2007

MUSCLE STRENGTH

Muscle Motion	Muscle	Nerve	Nerve Root
Elbow extension	Triceps	Radial	C6–C8

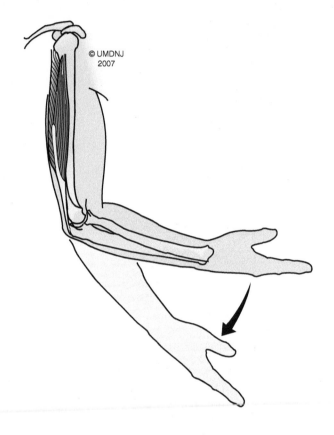

© UMDNJ
2007

Muscle Motion	Muscle	Nerve	Nerve Root
Wrist flexion	Flexor carpi radialis	Radial	C6–C7
Wrist flexion	Flexor carpi ulnaris	Ulnar	C7–T1

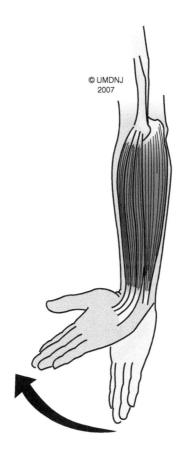

© UMDNJ
2007

MUSCLE STRENGTH

Muscle Motion	Muscle	Nerve	Nerve Root
Wrist extension	Extensor carpi radialis	Radial	C6–C7

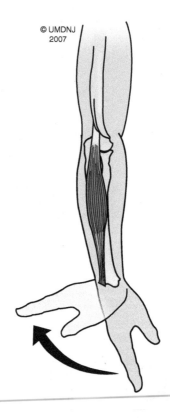

© UMDNJ
2007

Muscle Motion	Muscle	Nerve	Nerve Root
Finger abduction	Dorsal interossei	Ulnar	C8–T1

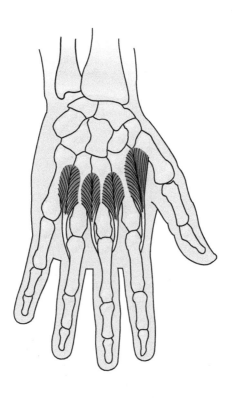

Muscle Motion	Muscle	Nerve	Nerve Root
Finger adduction	Palmar interossei	Ulnar	C8–T1

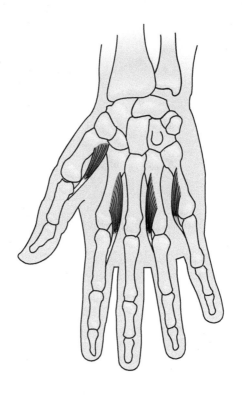

MUSCLE STRENGTH

LOWER EXTREMITY

Muscle Motion	Muscle	Nerve	Nerve Root
Foot dorsiflexion	Tibialis anterior	Deep peroneal	L4–L5

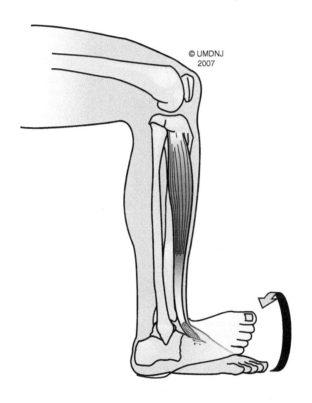

© UMDNJ
2007

Muscle Motion	Muscle	Nerve	Nerve Root
Foot eversion	Peroneus longus	Superficial peroneal	L5–S1

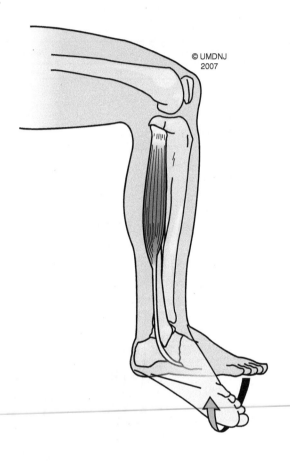

© UMDNJ
2007

CRANIAL HOLDS

CV4 HOLD

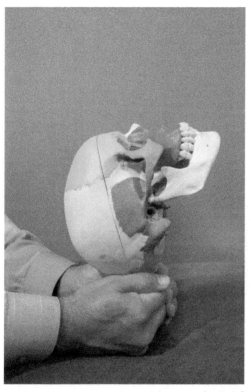

(continued)

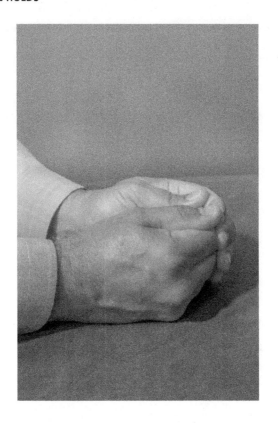

FRONTAL OCCIPITAL HOLD

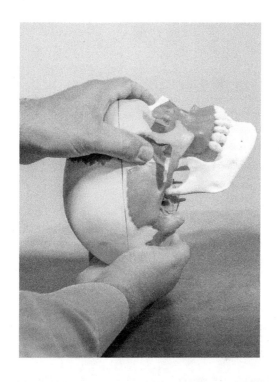

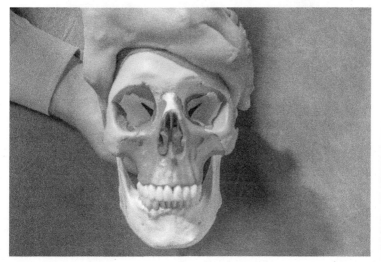

CRANIAL HOLDS

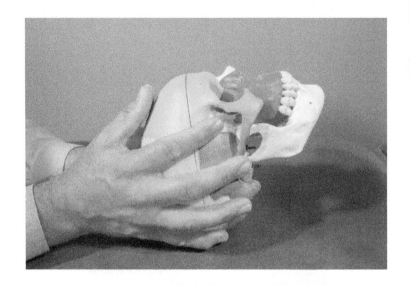

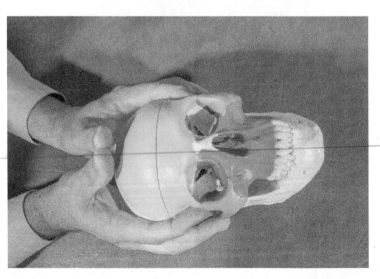

CRANIAL DIAGNOSIS

Flexion Phase[a]	
Sphenobasilar synchondrosis	Superior
Left sphenoid wing	Inferior and anterior
Right sphenoid wing	Inferior and anterior
Left occiput	Inferior and posterior
Right occiput	Inferior and posterior

[a]Adapted from Essig-Beatty, D. R., & Steele K. M. (2006). *The Pocket Manual of OMT: Osteopathic Manipulative Treatment for Physicians.* Philadelphia, PA: Lippincott Williams & Wilkins.

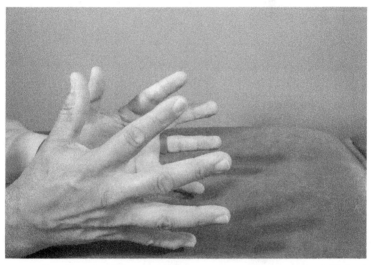

(Continued)

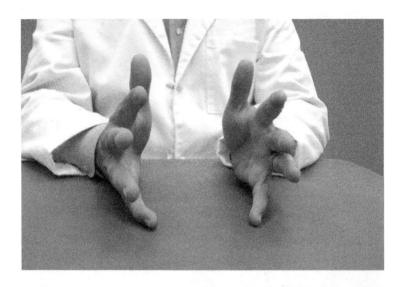

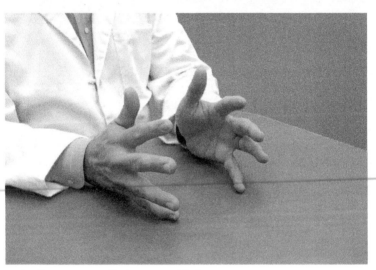

Hand positions are exaggerated for demonstration of the diagnosis.

Extension Phase	
Sphenobasilar synchondrosis	Inferior
Left sphenoid wing	Superior and posterior
Right sphenoid wing	Superior and posterior
Left occiput	Superior and anterior
Right occiput	Superior and anterior

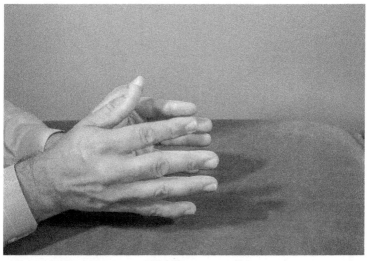

(Continued)

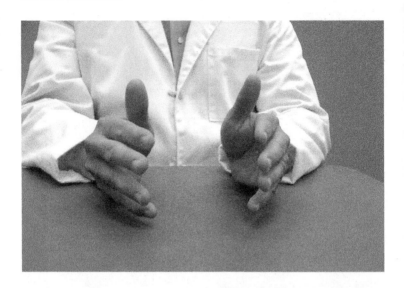

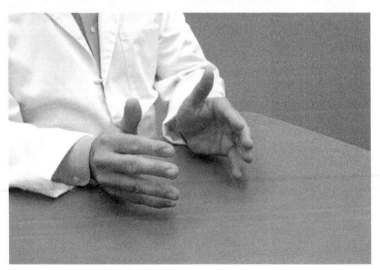

Hand positions are exaggerated for demonstration of the diagnosis.

CRANIAL DIAGNOSIS[1]

Left Lateral Strain[a]	
Right sphenoid wing	Lateral and posterior
Left sphenoid wing	Medial and anterior
Right occiput	Medial and posterior
Left occiput	Lateral and anterior

[a]Adapted from Essig-Beatty, D. R., & Steele K. M. (2006). *The Pocket Manual of OMT: Osteopathic Manipulative Treatment for Physician.* Philadelphia, PA: Lippincott Williams & Wilkins.

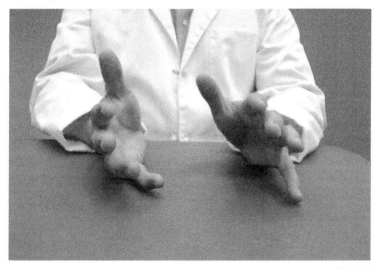

(Continued)

[1]*Strains are named for the direction of the sphenobasilar synchondrosis.*

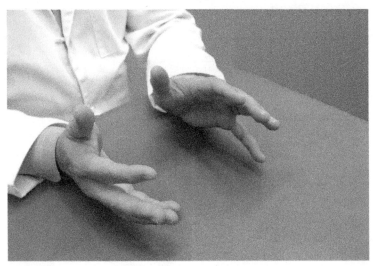

Hand positions are exaggerated for demonstration of the diagnosis.

Right Lateral Strain

Right sphenoid wing	Medial and anterior
Left sphenoid wing	Lateral and posterior
Right occiput	Lateral and anterior
Left occiput	Medial and posterior

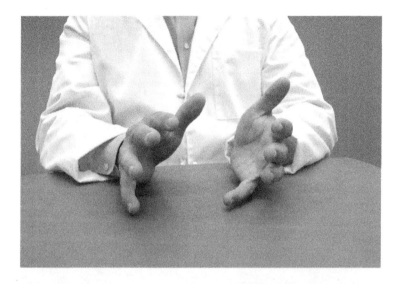

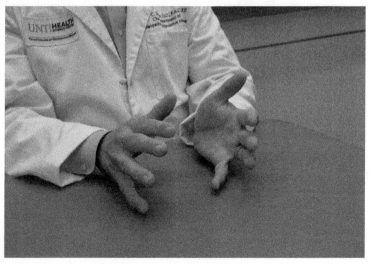

Hand positions are exaggerated for demonstration of the diagnosis.

CRANIAL DIAGNOSIS

CRANIAL DIAGNOSIS[2]

Left Torsion[a]	
Right sphenoid wing	Inferior
Left sphenoid wing	Superior
Right occiput	Superior
Left occiput	Inferior

[a]Adapted from Essig-Beatty, D. R., & Steele K. M. (2006). *The Pocket Manual of OMT: Osteopathic Manipulative Treatment for Physician*. Philadelphia, PA: Lippincott Williams & Wilkins.

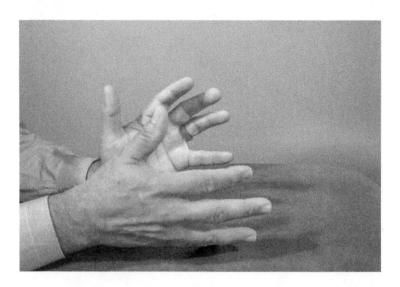

[2]Torsions are named for the superior greater wing of the sphenoid.

Right Torsion	
Right sphenoid wing	Superior
Left sphenoid wing	Inferior
Right occiput	Inferior
Left occiput	Superior

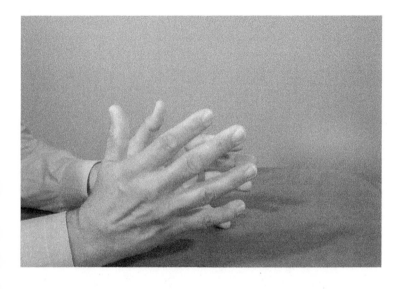

CRANIAL DIAGNOSIS

CRANIAL DIAGNOSIS[3]

Left Sidebending Rotation[a]	
Right sphenoid wing	Superior and posterior
Left sphenoid wing	Inferior and anterior
Right occiput	Superior and anterior
Left occiput	Inferior and posterior

[a]Adapted from Essig-Beatty, D. R., & Steele K. M. (2006). *The Pocket Manual of OMT: Osteopathic Manipulative Treatment for Physician*. Philadelphia, PA: Lippincott Williams & Wilkins.

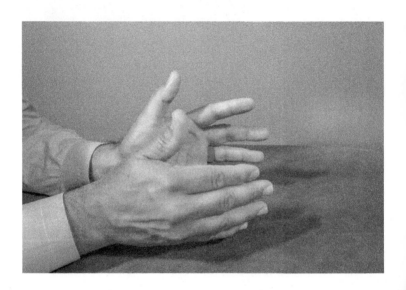

Right Sidebending Rotation

Right sphenoid wing	Inferior and anterior
Left sphenoid wing	Superior and posterior
Right occiput	Inferior and posterior
Left occiput	Superior and anterior

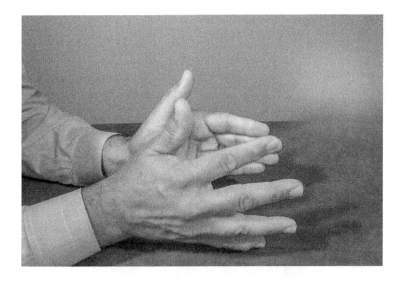

CRANIAL DIAGNOSIS[4]

Inferior Shear[a]	
Right sphenoid wing	Superior
Left sphenoid wing	Superior
Right occiput	Inferior
Left occiput	Inferior

[a]Adapted from Essig-Beatty, D. R., & Steele K. M. (2006). *The Pocket Manual of OMT: Osteopathic Manipulative Treatment for Physician*. Philadelphia, PA: Lippincott Williams & Wilkins.

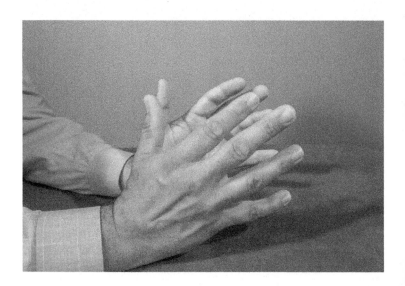

[4]Shears (vertical strains) are named for the direction of the basisphenoid movement.

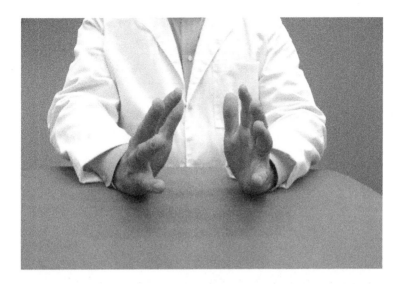

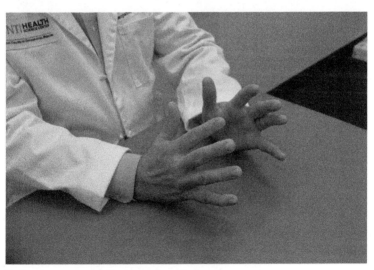

Hand positions are exaggerated for demonstration of the diagnosis.

CRANIAL DIAGNOSIS

Superior Shear	
Right sphenoid wing	Inferior
Left sphenoid wing	Inferior
Right occiput	Superior
Left occiput	Superior

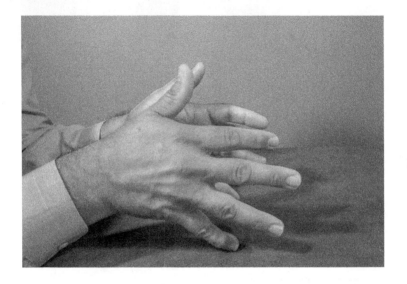

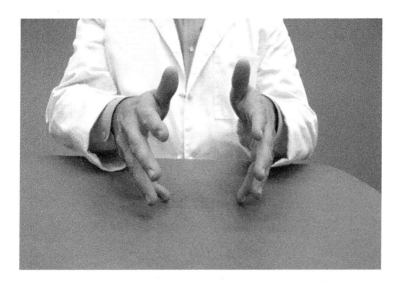

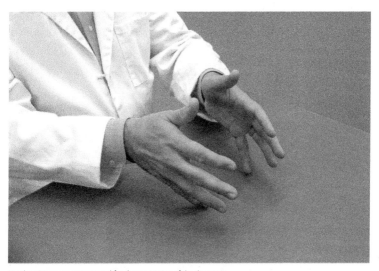

Hand positions are exaggerated for demonstration of the diagnosis.

SACRAL DIAGNOSIS

KEY POINTS TO REMEMBER IN SACRAL DIAGNOSIS

- The seated flexion test determines the abnormal side of sacral motion only.
- The oblique axis is opposite to the positive seated flexion test and is the normal side of sacral motion.

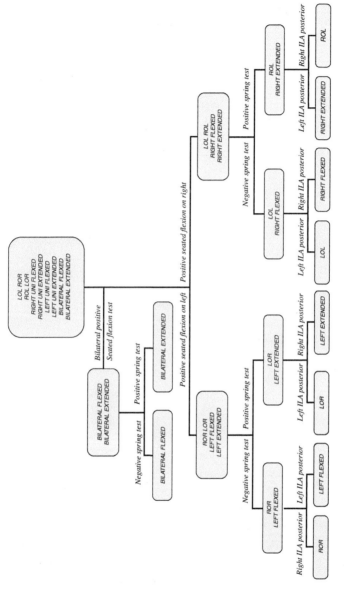

SACRAL DIAGNOSIS

SACRAL SOMATIC DYSFUNCTION DIAGNOSIS

LOL ROR
ROL LOR
RIGHT UNI FLEXED
RIGHT UNI EXTENDED
LEFT UNI FLEXED
LEFT UNI EXTENDED
BILATERAL FLEXED
BILATERAL EXTENDED

Bilateral positive Seated flexion test

BILATERAL FLEXED BILATERAL EXTENDED

Positive spring test → BILATERAL EXTENDED

Negative spring test → BILATERAL FLEXED

Positive seated flexion on left

ROR LOR
LEFT FLEXED
LEFT EXTENDED

Negative spring test → ROR LEFT FLEXED

- *Right ILA posterior* → ROR
- *Left ILA posterior* → LEFT FLEXED

Positive spring test → LOR LEFT EXTENDED

- *Left ILA posterior* → LOR
- *Right ILA posterior* → LEFT EXTENDED

Positive seated flexion on right

LOL ROL
RIGHT FLEXED
RIGHT EXTENDED

Negative spring test → LOL RIGHT FLEXED

- *Left ILA posterior* → LOL
- *Right ILA posterior* → RIGHT FLEXED

Positive spring test → ROL RIGHT EXTENDED

- *Left ILA posterior* → RIGHT EXTENDED
- *Right ILA posterior* → ROL

REFERENCES

REFERENCES

Low Back Pain	6, 7, 39, 50, 63, 83, 92, 93, 95, 96, 150,154
Medial Epicondylitis	89, 100, 140
Otitis Media/Serous/Infectious	34, 105, 138, 139
Pelvic Inflammatory Disease	6, 63
Peptic Ulcer Disease	6, 63, 88
Pharyngitis/Tonsillitis	6, 123, 128
Pneumonia	6, 15, 43, 56, 63, 75, 88, 110, 111, 112, 134, 141, 151, 156
Postconcussive Syndrome	63, 97
Pregnancy	6, 27, 28, 43, 63, 68, 84, 88, 91, 94, 141, 147
Premenstrual Syndrome	6, 43, 63
Pyloric Stenosis	6, 63, 88
Restless Legs Syndrome	18, 36, 118
Rhinitis, Allergic	6, 43, 63, 88
Sacroiliitis	18, 83, 92, 93, 95, 96
Sciatica	18, 20, 83, 92, 93, 95, 96
Scoliosis	6, 43, 63, 152
Sinusitis	6, 43, 63, 88, 123, 128, 131, 141
Spinal Stenosis	7, 30, 50, 53, 83, 92, 93, 95, 96
Tachycardia	43, 56, 60, 63, 81
Temporomandibular Joint Dysfunction	21, 40, 101
Thoracic Outlet Syndrome	6, 45, 63, 129, 146
Tinnitus	6
Torticollis	6, 43, 63, 117, 155
Urinary Tract Infection	6, 63, 88, 137
Vertigo/Labyrinthitis	25

1. Abbott, J. H., et al. (2013). Manual therapy, exercise therapy, or both, in addition to usual care, for osteoarthritis of the hip or knee: A randomized controlled trial. 1: Clinical effectiveness. *Osteoarthritis and Cartilage, 21*, (4), 525–234.
2. Ahmad, D., et al. (2014). Outcome of manipulation under anaesthesia in adhesive capsulitis patients. *Journal of the College of Physicians and Surgeons—Pakistan: JCPSP, 24*, (4), 293–294.
3. Ajimsha, M. (2011). Effectiveness of direct vs indirect technique myofascial release in the management of tension-type headache. *Journal of Bodywork and Movement Therapies, 15*, (4), 431–435.
4. Alexander, J. (2016). Resolution of new daily persistent headache after osteopathic manipulative treatment. *Journal of the American Osteopathic Association, 116*, (3), 182–185.
5. Alix, M. E., & Bates, D. K. (1999). A proposed etiology of cervicogenic headache: The neurophysiologic basis and anatomic relationship between the dura mater and the rectus posterior capitis minor muscle. *Journal of Manipulative and Physiological Therapeutics, 22*, (8), 534–539.
6. American Osteopathic Association. (2011). *Foundations of osteopathic medicine* (3rd ed.). Philadelphia, PA: Lippincott Williams and Wilkins.

Diagnosis	Page(s)
Allergy/Postnasal Drip	994,996
Ankle Sprain	612–617, 761
Anxiety	289,290,309
Arthritis (Inflammatory)	956
Arthritis (Osteoarthritis)	955–956, 1013
Asthma	883–887
Atelectasis	n/a
Bell's Palsy	511
Carpal Tunnel Syndrome	657, 805–807
Cervical Spondylosis	520
Cholecystitis	n/a
Chronic Obstructive Pulmonary Disease	215–219, 931–937
Colic	300, 742
Common Cold	505–506
Complex Regional Pain Syndrome (Reflex Sympathetic Dystrophy)	806
Congestive Heart Failure	n/a
Constipation	n/a
Costochondritis	n/a
Depression	287–289, 903–907
Diarrhea	n/a
Dupuytren Contracture/Trigger Finger	n/a
Dysmenorrhea	n/a
Dyspareunia/Pelvic Pain	n/a
Dysphagia	n/a
Emesis	n/a
Erectile Dysfunction	n/a
Fibromyalgia	976–977
Frozen Shoulder	658
Gastritis/Gastroesophageal Reflux Disease/Dyspepsia	922–923
Headache	507–510, 923
Hiccups (Singultus)	n/a
Hypertension	n/a
Ileus	n/a

Continued AOA. (2011). *Foundations of osteopathic medicine* (3rd edition). Philadelphia, PA: Lippincott Williams and Wilkins.

Inflammatory Bowel Disease (Crohn's Disease or Ulcerative Colitis)	n/a
Influenza	n/a
Irritable Bowel Syndrome	n/a
Lateral Epicondylitis	658
Low Back Pain	542–544, 572–573, 967–972, 1006–1017
Medial Epicondylitis	n/a
Otitis Media/Serous/Infectious	511–512, 741, 920–921
Pelvic Inflammatory Disease	n/a
Peptic Ulcer Disease	n/a
Pharyngitis/Tonsillitis	921–922
Pneumonia	n/a
Postconcussive Syndrome	n/a
Pregnancy	969–970
Premenstrual Syndrome	n/a
Pyloric Stenosis	n/a
Restless Legs Syndrome	n/a
Rhinitis, Allergic	994, 996
Sacroiliitis	n/a
Sciatica	n/a
Scoliosis	467, 470–472, 1107
Sinusitis	506–507, 921
Spinal Stenosis	n/a
Tachycardia	n/a
Temporomandibular Joint Dysfunction	922
Thoracic Outlet Syndrome	658–659
Tinnitus	359, 362, 366, 492
Torticollis	525
Urinary Tract Infection	963
Vertigo/Labyrinthitis	498, 509

7. Andersson, G. B., et al. (1999). A comparison of osteopathic spinal manipulation with standard care for patients with low back pain. *New England Journal of Medicine, 341*, (19), 1426–1431.

8. Attali, T. V., et al. (2013). Treatment of refractory irritable bowel syndrome with visceral osteopathy: Short-term and long-term results of a randomized trial. *Journal of Digestive Diseases, 14*, (12), 654–661.

9. Baltazar, G. A., et al. (2013). Effect of osteopathic manipulative treatment on incidence of postoperative ileus and hospital length of stay in general surgical patients. *Journal of the American Osteopathic Association, 113*, (3), 204–209.

10. Beal, M. C. (1983). Palpatory testing for somatic dysfunction in patients with cardiovascular disease. *Journal of the American Osteopathic Association, 82*, (11), 822–831.

11. Beal, M. C., & Morlock, J. W. (1984). Somatic dysfunction associated with pulmonary disease. *Journal of the American Osteopathic Association, 84*, 179–183.

12. Biondi, D. M. (2005). Physical treatments for headache: A structured review. *Headache, 45*, (6), 738–746.

13. Blood, S. D. (1980). Treatment of the sprained ankle. *Journal of the American Osteopathic Association, 79*, (11), 680–692.

14. Blood, S. D. (1986). The craniosacral mechanism and the tempermandibular joint. *Journal of the American Osteopathic Association, 86*, (8), 512–519.

15. Bockenhauer, S. E., et al. (2002). Quantifiable effects of osteopathic manipulative techniques on patients with chronic asthma. *Journal of the American Osteopathic Association, 102*, (7), 371–375.

16. Boesler, D., et al. (1993). Efficacy of high-velocity low-amplitude manipulative technique in subjects with low-back pain during menstrual cramping. *Journal of the American Osteopathic Association, 93*, (2), 203–214.

17. Bordoni, B., & Marelli, F. (2015). The fascial system and exercise intolerance in patients with chronic heart failure: Hypothesis of osteopathic treatment. *Journal of Multidisciplinary Healthcare, 8*, 489–494.

18. Boyajian-O'Neill, L. A., et al. (2008). Diagnosis and management of piriformis syndrome: An osteopathic approach. *Journal of the American Osteopathic Association, 108*, (11), 657–664.

19. Brantingham, J. W., et al. (2011). Manipulative therapy for shoulder pain and disorders: Expansion of a systematic review. *Journal of Manipulative and Physiological Therapeutics, 34*, (5), 314–346.

20. Brantingham, J. W., et al. (2012). Manipulative therapy for lower extremity conditions: Update of a literature review. *Journal of Manipulative and Physiological Therapeutics, 35*, (2), 127–166.

21. Brantingham, J. W., et al. (2013). Manipulative and multimodal therapy for upper extremity and temporomandibular disorders: A systematic review. *Journal of Manipulative and Physiological Therapeutics, 36*, (3), 143–201.

22. Bromley, D. (2014). Abdominal massage in the management of chronic constipation for children with disability. *Community Practitioner, 87*, (12), 25–29.

23. Bronfort, G., et al. (2001). Efficacy of spinal manipulation on chronic headache: A systemic review. *Journal of Manipulative and Physiological Therapeutics, 24*, (7), 457–466.

24. Brugman, R., et al. (2010). The effect of osteopathic treatment on chronic constipation: A pilot study. *International Journal of Osteopathic Medicine, 13*, (1), 17–23.

25. Burmeister, D. B., et al. (2010). Management of benign paroxysmal positional vertigo with the canalith repositioning maneuver in the emergency department setting. *Journal of the American Osteopathic Association, 110*, (10), 602–604.

26. Burnham, T., et al. (2015). Effectiveness of osteopathic manipulative treatment for carpal tunnel syndrome: A pilot project. *Journal of the American Osteopathic Association, 115*, (3), 138–148.

27. Carpenter, S., & Woolley, A. (2001). Osteopathic manipulative treatment of low back pain during labor. *The AAO Journal: A Publication of the American Academy of Osteopathy, 11*, (3), 21–23.

28. Cassidy, I. T., & Jones, C. G. (2002). A retrospective case report of symphysis pubis dysfunction in a pregnant woman. *Journal of Osteopathic Medicine, 5*, (2), 83–86.

29. Castien, R. F., et al. (2011). Effectiveness of manual therapy for chronic tension-type headache: A pragmatic, randomised, clinical trial. *Cephalalgia, 31*, (2), 133–143.

30. Celenay, S. T., et al. (2016). Cervical and scapulothoracic stabilization exercises with and without connective tissue massage for chronic mechanical neck pain: A prospective, randomised controlled trial. *Manual Therapy, 21*, 144, 150.

31. Cerritelli, F., et al. (2011). Osteopathic manipulation as a complementary treatment for the prevention of cardiac complications: 12-months follow-up of intima media and blood pressure on a cohort affected by hypertension. *Journal of Bodywork and Movement Therapies, 15*, (1), 68–74.

32. Chaibi, A., et al. (2011). Manual therapies for migraine: A systematic review. *The Journal of Headache and Pain, 12*, (2), 127–133.

33. Chaitow, L. (2005). Cranial manipulation (2nd ed.). Philadelphia, PA: Churchill-Livingston, Elsevier.

34. Channell, M. K. (2008). Modified Muncie technique: Osteopathic manipulation for eustachian tube dysfunction and illustrative report of case. *Journal of the American Osteopathic Association, 108*, (5), 260–263.

REFERENCES

35. Channell, M. K., et al. (2009). Management of chronic posttraumatic headache: A multidisciplinary approach. *Journal of the American Osteopathic Association*, *109*, (9), 509–513.

36. Collins, N., et al. (2009). Foot orthoses and physiotherapy in the treatment of patellofemoral pain syndrome: Randomised clinical trial. *British Journal of Sports Medicine*, *43*, (3), 169–171.

37. Crow, W. T., & Gorodinsky, L. (2009). Does osteopathic manipulative treatment (OMT) improves outcomes in patients who develop postoperative ileus: A retrospective chart review. *International Journal of Osteopathic Medicine*, *12*, (1), 32–37.

38. Crowell, M. S., & Tragord, B. S. (2015). Orthopaedic manual physical therapy for shoulder pain and impaired movement in a patient with glenohumeral joint osteoarthritis: A case report. *The Journal of Orthopaedic and Sports Physical Therapy*, *45*, (6), 453–461, A1–A3.

39. Cruser, D., et al. (2012). A randomized, controlled trial of osteopathic manipulative treatment for acute low back pain in active duty military personnel. *The Journal of Manual & Manipulative Therapy*, *20*, (1), 5–15.

40. Cuccia, A. M., et al. (2010). Osteopathic manual therapy versus conventional conservative therapy in the treatment of temporomandibular disorders: A randomized controlled trial. *Journal of Bodywork and Movement Therapies*, *14*, (2), 179–184.

41. da Silva, R. C., et al. (2013). Increase of lower esophageal sphincter pressure after osteopathic intervention on the diaphragm in patients with gastroesophageal reflux. *Diseases of the Esophagus*, *26*, (5), 451–456.

42. Dambro, M. (2004). *Griffith's 5-minute consult 2005*. Philadelphia, PA: Lippincott Williams and Wilkins.

43. DiGiovanna, E., et al. (2005). *An osteopathic approach to diagnosis and treatment* (3rd ed.). Philadelphia, PA: Lippincott Williams and Wilkins.

Diagnosis	Page(s)
Allergy/Postnasal Drip	n/a
Ankle Sprain	502–503, 519–522
Anxiety	n/a
Arthritis (Inflammatory)	466
Arthritis (Osteoarthritis)	466
Asthma	619–620
Atelectasis	n/a
Bell's Palsy	661–662
Carpal Tunnel Syndrome	465
Cervical Spondylosis	n/a
Cholecystitis	n/a
Chronic Obstructive Pulmonary Disease	620
Colic	637–638
Common Cold	n/a
Complex Regional Pain Syndrome (Reflex Sympathetic Dystrophy)	662–663
Congestive Heart Failure	627–629
Constipation	633
Costochondritis	n/a
Depression	n/a
Diarrhea	632–633
Dupuytren Contracture/Trigger Finger	465–466
Dysmenorrhea	646–651
Dyspareunia/Pelvic Pain	n/a
Dysphagia	631

Continued DiGiovanna, E., Schiowitz, S., & Dowling, D. (2005). *An osteopathic approach to diagnosis and treatment* (3rd ed.). Philadelphia, PA: Lippincott Williams and Wilkins.

Emesis	n/a
Erectile Dysfunction	n/a
Fibromyalgia	n/a
Frozen Shoulder	465
Gastritis/Gastroesophageal Reflux Disease/Dyspepsia	n/a
Headache	606–607
Hiccups (Singultus)	635
Hypertension	n/a
Ileus	633–635
Inflammatory Bowel Disease (Crohn's Disease or Ulcerative Colitis)	n/a
Influenza	589–591
Irritable Bowel Syndrome	633, 635–637
Lateral Epicondylitis	n/a
Low Back Pain	n/a
Medial Epicondylitis	n/a
Otitis Media/Serous/Infectious	n/a
Pelvic Inflammatory Disease	n/a
Peptic Ulcer Disease	n/a
Pharyngitis/Tonsillitis	n/a
Pneumonia	619
Postconcussive Syndrome	n/a
Pregnancy	651–657
Premenstrual Syndrome	646–651
Pyloric Stenosis	n/a
Restless Legs Syndrome	n/a
Rhinitis, Allergic	614
Sacroiliitis	n/a
Sciatica	n/a
Scoliosis	226–227
Sinusitis	170, 611–614
Spinal Stenosis	n/a
Tachycardia	627
Temporomandibular Joint Dysfunction	n/a
Thoracic Outlet Syndrome	n/a
Tinnitus	n/a
Torticollis	170–171
Urinary Tract Infection	n/a
Vertigo/Labyrinthitis	n/a

44. Diniz, L. R., et al. (2014). Qualitative evaluation of osteopathic manipulative therapy in a patient with gastroesophageal reflux disease: A brief report. *Journal of the American Osteopathic Association, 114*, (3), 180–188.
45. Dobrusin, R. (1989). An osteopathic approach to conservative management of thoracic outlet syndromes. *Journal of the American Osteopathic Association, 89*, (8), 1046–1057.
46. Dowling, D. (2000). Progressive inhibition of neuromuscular structures (PINS) technique. *Journal of the American Osteopathic Association, 100*, (5), 285–298.
47. Dugenhardt, B., & Kuchera, M. (2006). Osteopathic evaluation and manipulative treatment in reducing the morbidity of otitis media: A pilot study. *Journal of the American Osteopathic Association, 106*, (6), 327–334.

48. Dunning, J. R., et al. (2016). Upper cervical and upper thoracic manipulation versus mobilization and exercise in patients with cervicogenic headache: A multi-center randomized clinical trial. *BMC Musculoskeletal Disorders, 17*, 64.

49. Eisenhart, A. W., et al. (2003). Osteopathic manipulative treatment in the emergency department for patients with acute ankle injuries. *Journal of the American Osteopathic Association, 103*, (9), 417–421.

50. Ellestad, S. M., et al. (1988). Electromyographic and skin resistance responses to osteopathic manipulative treatment for low-back pain. *Journal of the American Osteopathic Association, 88*, (8), 991–997.

51. Florance, B. M., et al. (2012). Osteopathy improves the severity of irritable bowel syndrome: A pilot randomized sham-controlled study. *European Journal of Gastroenterology & Hepatology, 24*, (8), 944–999.

52. Flotildes, K. L., et. al. (2001). The evaluation of the effect of osteopathic manipulative techniques (OMT) on headache pain. *Journal of the American Osteopathic Association, 101*, 474.

53. Franke, H., et al. (2015). Osteopathic manipulative treatment for chronic nonspecific neck pain: A systematic review and meta-analysis. *International Journal of Osteopathic Medicine, 18*, (4), 255–267.

54. Freitag, F. (1983). Osteopathic treatment of migraine. *Osteopathic Annals, 11*, (6), 19–26.

55. Frobert, O., et al. (1999). Musculo-skeletal pathology in patients with angina pectoris and normal coronary angiograms. *Journal of Internal Medicine, 245*, 237–246.

56. Frymann, V. M. (1978). The osteopathic approach to cardiac and pulmonary problems. *Journal of the American Osteopathic Association, 77*, 668–673.

57. Gallagher, R. M. (2005). Headache pain. *Journal of the American Osteopathic Association, 105*, (9 suppl 4), S7–11.

58. Gallego, P. H., et al. (2007). Indirect influence of specific Kaltenborn glide mobilizations of the carpal joint on a subject with neurological impairments. *Journal of Bodywork and Movement Therapies, 11*, (4), 275–284.

59. Gamber, R., et. al. (2002). Osteopathic manipulative treatment in conjunction with medication relieves pain associated with fibromyalgia syndrome: Results of a randomized clinical pilot project. *Journal of the American Osteopathic Association, 102*, (6), 321–325.

60. Giles, P. D., et al. (2013). Suboccipital decompression enhances heart rate variability indices of cardiac control in healthy subjects. *Journal of Alternative and Complementary Medicine (New York, N.Y.), 19*, (2), 92–96.

61. Guiney, P., et. al. (2005). Effects of osteopathic manipulative treatment on pediatric patients with asthma: A randomized controlled trial. *Journal of the American Osteopathic Association, 105*, (1), 7–12.

62. Gürsen, C., et al. (2015). Effect of connective tissue manipulation on symptoms and quality of life in patients with chronic constipation: A randomized controlled trial. *Journal of Manipulative and Physiological Therapeutics, 35*, (5), 335–343.

63. Guyton, A. C., & Hall, J. E. (2006). *Textbook of medical physiology* (11th ed.). Philadelphia, PA: Elsevier Saunders.

64. Hack, G. D., et al. (1995). Anatomic relation between the rectus capitis posterior minor muscle and dura mater. *Spine, 20*, (23), 2484–2486.

65. Hains, G., & Hains, F. (2000). Combined ischemic compression and spinal manipulation in the treatment of fibromyalgia: A preliminary estimate dose and efficacy. *Journal of Manipulative and Physiological Therapeutics, 23*, (4), 225–230.

66. Hanten, W. P., et al. (2001). The effectiveness of CV-4 and resting position techniques on subjects with tension-type headaches. [Abstract. Reprint from the Journal of Manual & Manipulative Therapy, 1999, 7, (2), 64–70.] *Journal of Osteopathic Medicine, 4*, (2), 62.

67. Heineman, K. (2014). Osteopathic manipulative treatment in the management of biliary dyskinesia. *Journal of the American Osteopathic Association, 114,* (2), 129–133.

68. Hensel, K. L., et al. (2015). Pregnancy Research on Osteopathic Manipulation Optimizing Treatment Effects: The PROMOTE study. *American Journal of Obstetrics and Gynecology, 212,* (1), 108.e1–108.e9.

69. Hermann, E. (1965). Postoperative adynamic ileus: Its prevention and treatment by osteopathic manipulation. *The DO, 6,* (2), 163–164.

70. Hitchcock, M. E. (1976). The manipulative approach to the management of primary dysmenorrhea. *Journal of the American Osteopathic Association, 75,* 909–918.

71. Hoag, J. M. (1972). Musculoskeletal involvement in chronic lung disease. *Journal of the American Osteopathic Association, 71,* 698–706.

72. Howell, J. N., et al. (2006). Stretch reflex and Hoffmann reflex responses to osteopathic manipulative treatment in subjects with Achilles tendinitis. *Journal of the American Osteopathic Association, 106,* (9), 537–545.

73. Howell, R., et al. (1975). The influence of osteopathic manipulative therapy in the management of patients with chronic obstructive lung disease. *Journal of the American Osteopathic Association, 74,* 757–760.

74. Hoyt, W. H., et al. (1979). Osteopathic manipulation in the treatment of muscle-contraction headache. *Journal of the American Osteopathic Association, 78,* 322–325.

75. Hruby, R. J., & Hoffman, K. N. (2007). Avian influenza: An osteopathic component to treatment. *Osteopathic Medicine and Primary Care, 1,* 10.

76. Hundscheid, H. W., et al. (2007). Treatment of irritable bowel syndrome with osteopathy: Results of a randomized controlled pilot study. *Journal of Gastroenterology and Hepatology, 22,* (9), 1394–1398.

77. Jacobson, E., et al. (1989). Shoulder pain and repetition strain injury to the supraspinatus muscle: Etiology and manipulative treatment. *Journal of the American Osteopathic Association, 89, (8),* 1037–1045.

78. Jardine, W. M., et al. (2012). The effect of osteopathic manual therapy on the vascular supply to the lower extremity in individuals with knee osteoarthritis: A randomized trial. *International Journal of Osteopathic Medicine, 15,* (4), 125–133.

79. Johnson, F. (1972). Some observations on the use of osteopathic therapy in the care of patients with cardiac disease. *Journal of the American Osteopathic Association, 71,* 799–804.

80. Juberg, M., et al. (2015). Pilot study of massage in veterans with knee osteoarthritis. *Journal of Alternative and Complementary Medicine (New York, N.Y.), 21,* (6), 333–338.

81. Julian, M. R. (2008). Treatment of paroxysmal supraventricular tachycardia using instrument-assisted manipulation of the fourth rib: A 6-year case study. *Journal of Manipulative and Physiological Therapeutics, 31,* (5), 389–391.

82. Jull, G., et al. (2002). A randomized controlled trial of exercise and manipulative therapy for cervicogenic headache. *Spine, 27,* (17), 1835–1843.

83. Kappler, R. E. (1973). Role of psoas mechanism in low-back complaints. *Journal of the American Osteopathic Association, 72,* 794–801.

84. King, H. H. (2000). Osteopathic manipulative treatment in prenatal care: Evidence supporting improved outcomes and health policy implications. *The AAO Journal: A Publication of the American Academy of Osteopathy, 10,* (2), 25–33.

85. Knebl, J., et al. (2002). Improving functional ability in the elderly via the Spencer technique, an osteopathic manipulative treatment: A randomized control trial. *Journal of the American Osteopathic Association, 102,* (7), 387–396.

86. Knott, E. M., et al. (2005). Increased lymphatic flow in the thoracic duct during manipulative intervention. *Journal of the American Osteopathic Association, 105,* (10), 447–456.

REFERENCES

87. Kuchera, M. (2005). Osteopathic manipulative medicine considerations in patients with chronic pain. *Journal of the American Osteopathic Association*, *105*, (9), 529–536.
88. Kuchera, M., & Kuchera, W. (1994). *Osteopathic considerations in systemic dysfunction*. Columbus, OH: Greydon Press.

Diagnosis	Page(s)
Allergy/Postnasal Drip	n/a
Ankle Sprain	n/a
Anxiety	n/a
Arthritis (Inflammatory)	159–167
Arthritis (Osteoarthritis)	159–167
Asthma	48–50
Atelectasis	n/a
Bell's Palsy	n/a
Carpal Tunnel Syndrome	n/a
Cervical Spondylosis	n/a
Cholecystitis	n/a
Chronic Obstructive Pulmonary Disease	39, 48
Colic	172
Common Cold	15, 17–18, 31
Complex Regional Pain Syndrome (Reflex Sympathetic Dystrophy)	n/a
Congestive Heart Failure	56, 66, 185, 232
Constipation	97, 98, 104, 105
Costochondritis	58
Depression	n/a
Diarrhea	97–98, 104–105
Dupuytren Contracture/Trigger Finger	186
Dysmenorrhea	139–141
Dyspareunia/Pelvic Pain	n/a
Dysphagia	n/a
Emesis	104–105
Erectile Dysfunction	142–143
Fibromyalgia	167
Frozen Shoulder	n/a
Gastritis/Gastroesophageal Reflux Disease/Dyspepsia	n/a
Headache	44, 104–105
Hiccups (Singultus)	n/a
Hypertension	61–66
Ileus	100–104, 198–199
Inflammatory Bowel Disease (Crohn's Disease or Ulcerative Colitis)	n/a
Influenza	n/a
Irritable Bowel Syndrome	109–121
Lateral Epicondylitis	n/a
Low Back Pain	n/a
Medial Epicondylitis	n/a
Otitis Media/Serous/Infectious	4–15
Pelvic Inflammatory Disease	n/a
Peptic Ulcer Disease	86–87
Pharyngitis/Tonsillitis	n/a
Pneumonia	40–46

Continued Kuchera, M., & Kuchera, W. (1994). *Osteopathic considerations in systemic dysfunction*. Columbus, OH: Greydon Press.

Postconcussive Syndrome	n/a
Pregnancy	149–158
Premenstrual Syndrome	n/a
Pyloric Stenosis	79–93
Restless Legs Syndrome	n/a
Rhinitis, Allergic	15–18, 31
Sacroiliitis	n/a
Sciatica	n/a
Scoliosis	n/a
Sinusitis	12, 15, 18
Spinal Stenosis	n/a
Tachycardia	n/a
Temporomandibular Joint Dysfunction	n/a
Thoracic Outlet Syndrome	n/a
Tinnitus	n/a
Torticollis	n/a
Urinary Tract Infection	134–135
Vertigo/Labyrinthitis	n/a

89. Küçükşen, S., et al. (2013). Muscle energy technique versus corticosteroid injection for management of chronic lateral epicondylitis: Randomized controlled trial with 1-year follow-up. *Archives of Physical Medicine and Rehabilitation*, *94*, (11), 2068–2074.

90. Lancaster, D. G., & Crow, W. T. (2006). Osteopathic manipulative treatment of a 26-year-old woman with Bell's palsy. *Journal of the American Osteopathic Association*, *106*, (5), 285–289.

91. Licciardone, J. C., & Aryal, S. (2013). Prevention of progressive back-specific dysfunction during pregnancy: An assessment of osteopathic manual treatment based on Cochrane Back Review Group criteria. *Journal of the American Osteopathic Association*, 113, (10), 728–736.

92. Licciardone, J. C., & Aryal, S. (2014). Clinical response and relapse in patients with chronic low back pain following osteopathic manual treatment: Results from the OSTEOPATHIC trial. *Manual Therapy*, *19*, (6), 541–548.

93. Licciardone, J. C., et al. (2003). Osteopathic manipulative treatment for chronic low back pain: A randomized controlled trial. *Spine*, *28*, (13), 1355–1362.

94. Licciardone, J. C., et al. (2010). Osteopathic manipulative treatment of back pain and related symptoms during pregnancy: A randomized controlled trial. *American Journal of Obstetrics and Gynecology*, *202*, (1), 43.e1–43.e8.

95. Licciardone, J. C., et al. (2013). Outcomes of osteopathic manual treatment for chronic low back pain according to baseline pain severity: Results from the OSTEOPATHIC trial. *Manual Therapy*, *18*, (6), 533–540.

96. Licciardone, J. C., et al. (2016). Recovery from chronic low back pain after osteopathic manipulative treatment: A randomized controlled trial. *Journal of the American Osteopathic Association*, *116*, (3), 144–155.

97. Magoun, H. (1966). *Osteopathy in the cranial field* (3rd ed.). Indianapolis, IN: The Cranial Academy.

98. Mall, R. (1973). An evaluation of routine pulmonary function tests as indicators of responsiveness of a patient with chronic obstructive lung disease to osteopathic health care. *Journal of the American Osteopathic Association*, *73*, 327–333.

99. Mannino, J. R. (1979). The application of neurologic reflexes to the treatment of hypertension. *Journal of the American Osteopathic Association*, *79*, (4), 225–231.

REFERENCES

100. Marcolino, A. M., et al. (2016). Multimodal approach to rehabilitation of the patients with lateral epicondylosis: A case series. *SpringerPlus*, *5*, (1), 1718.

101. Martins, W. R., et al. (2016). Efficacy of musculoskeletal manual approach in the treatment of temporomandibular joint disorder: A systematic review with meta-analysis. *Manual Therapy*, *21*, 10–17.

102. McPartland, J., et al. (2005). Cannabimimetic effects of osteopathic manipulative treatment. *Journal of the American Osteopathic Association*, *105*, (6), 283–291.

103. Menck, J. Y., et al (2000). Thoracic spine dysfunction in upper extremity complex regional pain syndrome. [Abstract. Reprint from the Journal of Orthopaedic & Sports Physical Therapy, 2000, 30, (7), 401–409.] *Journal of Osteopathic Medicine*, *4*, (2), 71.

104. Mesa-Jiménez, J., et al. (2015). Multimodal manual therapy vs. pharmacological care for management of tension type headache: A meta-analysis of randomized trials. *Cephalalgia*, *35*, (14), 1323–1332.

105. Mills, M. V., et al. (2003). The use of osteopathic manipulative treatment as adjuvant therapy in children with recurrent acute otitis media. *Archives of Pediatrics & Adolescent Medicine*, *157*, (9), 861–866.

106. Molins-Cubero, S., et al. (2014). Changes in pain perception after pelvis manipulation in women with primary dysmenorrhea: A randomized controlled trial. *Pain Medicine (Malden, Mass.)*, *15*, (9), 1455–1463.

107. Moore, K., et al. (2006). *Essential clinical anatomy*. Philadelphia, PA: Lippincott Williams and Wilkins.

108. Morley, T. F. (2003). Osteopathic manipulative therapy (OMT) as a non-pharmacological treatment for stable patients with emphysema and chronic bronchitis. *Journal of the American Osteopathic Association*, *103*, (8).

109. Müller, A., et al. (2014). Effectiveness of osteopathic manipulative therapy for managing symptoms of irritable bowel syndrome: A systematic review. *Journal of the American Osteopathic Association*, *114*, (6), 470–479.

110. Noll, D. R., et al. (2000). Benefits of osteopathic manipulative treatment for hospitalized elderly patients with pneumonia. *Journal of the American Osteopathic Association*, *100*, (12), 776–782.

111. Noll, D. R., et al. (2016). Multicenter osteopathic pneumonia study in the elderly: Subgroup analysis on hospital length of stay, ventilator-dependent respiratory failure rate, and in-hospital mortality rate. *Journal of the American Osteopathic Association*, *116*, (9), 574–587.

112. Noll, D. R., et al. (1999). Adjunctive osteopathic manipulative treatment in the elderly hospitalized with pneumonia: A pilot study. *Journal of the American Osteopathic Association*, *99*, (3), 143–152.

113. Northrup, T. L. (1961). Manipulative management of hypertension. *Journal of the American Osteopathic Association*, *60*, 973–978.

114. Olds, K., & Berkowitz, M. R. (2012) Isolated calcaneofibular ligament injuries treated with osteopathic manipulative treatment: A case series. *International Journal of Osteopathic Medicine*, *15*, (4), 166–172.

115. Osborne, G. G. (1994). Manual medicine and its role in psychiatry. *The AAO Journal: A Publication of the American Academy of Osteopath*, *4*, (1), 16–21.

116. O-Yurvati, A., et al. (2005). Hemodynamic effects of osteopathic manipulative treatment immediately after coronary artery bypass surgery. *Journal of the American Osteopathic Association*, *105*, (10), 475–481.

117. Paul, F., & Buser, B. (1996). Osteopathic manipulative treatment applications for the emergency department patient. *Journal of the American Osteopathic Association*, *96*, (7), 403–409.

118. Peters, P., et al. (2013). Counterstrain manipulation in the treatment of restless legs syndrome: A pilot singleblind randomized controlled trial; the CARL trial. *International Musculoskeletal Medicine*, *34*, (4), 136–140.

119. Pintal, W., & Kurtz, M. (1989). An integrated osteopathic treatment approach in acute otitis media. *Journal of the American Osteopathic Association, 89, (9)*, 1139–1141.

120. Plotkin, B. J., et al. (2001). Adjunctive osteopathic manipulative treatment in women with depression: A pilot study. *Journal of the American Osteopathic Association, 101*, (9), 517–523.

121. Pratt-Harrington, D. (2000). Galbreath technique: A manipulative treatment for otitis media revisited. *Journal of the American Osteopathic Association, 100*, (10), 635–639.

122. Pratt-Harrington, D., & Neptune-Ceran, R. (1995). The effect of osteopathic manipulative treatment in the post abdominal surgical patient. *The American Academy of Osteopathy Journal, 5*, (3), 9–13.

123. Purse, F. M. (1966). Manipulative therapy of upper respiratory infections in children. *Journal of the American Osteopathic Association, 65*, 964–972.

124. Pyszora, A., & Krajnik, M. (2010). The role of physiotherapy in palliative care for the relief of constipation: A case report. *Advances in Palliative Medicine, 9*, (2), 45–47.

125. Riley, G. W. (2000). Osteopathic success in the treatment of influenza and pneumonia. 1919. [Reprint from the Journal of the American Osteopathic Association, 1919.] *Journal of the American Osteopathic Association, 100*, (5), 315–319.

126. Rolle, G., et al. (2014). Pilot trial of osteopathic manipulative therapy for patients with frequent episodic tension-type headache. *Journal of the American Osteopathic Association, 114*, (9), 678–685.

127. Rowane, W., & Rowane, M. (1999). An osteopathic approach to asthma. *Journal of the American Osteopathic Association, 99*, (5), 259–264.

128. Schmidt, C. (1982). Osteopathic manipulative therapy as a primary factor of upper, middle, and pararespiratory infections. *Journal of the American Osteopathic Association, 81*, (6), 382–388.

129. Schuenke, M., et al. (2010). *Thieme atlas of anatomy: General anatomy and musculoskeletal system.* New York, NY: Thieme Medical.

130. Sholars, H. (1996). AAO case history: Common problems in newborns and infants. *The AAO Journal: A Publication of the American Academy of Osteopathy, 6*, (3), 19–20.

131. Shrum, K., et al. (2001). Sinusitis in children: The importance of diagnosis and treatment. *Journal of the American Osteopathic Association, 101*, (5), S8–S13.

132. Sinclair, M. (2011). The use of abdominal massage to treat chronic constipation. *Journal of Bodywork and Movement Therapies, 15*, (4), 436–445.

133. Siu, G., et al. (2012). Osteopathic manipulative medicine for carpal tunnel syndrome. *Journal of the American Osteopathic Association, 112*, (3), 127–139.

134. Sleszynski, S. L., & Kelso, A. F. (1993). Comparison of thoracic manipulation with incentive spirometry in preventing postoperative atelectasis. *Journal of the American Osteopathic Association, 93*, (8), 834–845.

135. Snider, K. T. (2016). The use of osteopathic manipulative treatment as part of an integrated treatment for infantile colic: A case report. *AAO Journal, 26*, (2), 15–18.

136. Spiegel, A. J., et al. (2003). Osteopathic manipulative medicine in the treatment of hypertension: An alternative, conventional approach. *Heart Disease, 5*, (4), 272–278.

137. Stark, E. H. (1975). Evaluation and management of urinary tract infections. *Osteopathic Annals*, 34–40.

138. Steele, K. M., et al. (2010). Brief report of a clinical trial on the duration of middle ear effusion in young children using a standardized osteopathic manipulative medicine protocol. *Journal of the American Osteopathic Association, 110*, (5), 278–284.

139. Steele, K. M., et al. (2014). Effect of osteopathic manipulative treatment on middle ear effusion following acute otitis media in young children: A pilot study. *Journal of the American Osteopathic Association, 114*, (6), 436–447.

140. Steiner, C. (1976). Tennis elbow. *Journal of the American Osteopathic Association, 75*, (6), 575–581.

REFERENCES

141. Stiles, E. G. (1979). Osteopathic manipulation in a hospital environment. *Journal of the American Osteopathic Association, 76*, 243–258.
142. Stoll, S. T, & Simmons, S. L. (2000). Inpatient rehabilitation and manual medicine. *Physical Medicine and Rehabilitation: State of the Art Reviews, 14*, (1), 85–106.
143. Stuhr, S. H., et al. (2014). Use of orthopedic manual physical therapy to manage chronic orofacial pain and tension-type headache in an adolescent. *The Journal of Manual & Manipulative Therapy, 22*, (1), 51–58.
144. Sucher, B. (1993). Myofascial release of carpal tunnel syndrome. *Journal of the American Osteopathic Association, 93*, (1), 92–101.
145. Sucher, B. (1993). Myofascial release of carpal tunnel syndrome: Documentation with magnetic resonance imaging. *Journal of the American Osteopathic Association, 93*, (12), 1273–1278.
146. Sucher, B. (1995). Palpatory diagnosis and manipulative management of carpal tunnel syndrome: Part 2, "double crush" and thoracic outlet syndrome. *Journal of the American Osteopathic Association, 95*, (8), 471–479.
147. Taylor, G. W. (1949). The osteopathic management of nausea and vomiting of pregnancy. *Journal of the American Osteopathic Association, 48*, (11), 581–582.
148. Torsten, L. (2005). *Cranial osteopathy: Principles and practice*. London, United Kingdom: Churchill Livingstone.
149. Travell, J. G. (1977). A trigger point for hiccup. *Journal of the American Osteopathic Association, 77*, 308–312.
150. von Heymann, W. J., et al. (2013). Spinal high-velocity low amplitude manipulation in acute nonspecific low back pain: A double-blinded randomized controlled trial in comparison with diclofenac and placebo. *Spine (Phila Pa 1976), 38*, (7), 540–548.
151. Washington, K., et al. (2003). Presence of Chapman reflex points in hospitalized patients with pneumonia. *Journal of the American Osteopathic Association, 103*, (10), 479–483.
152. Weatherly, J. (1998). Scoliosis and osteopathic manipulative treatment. *The AAO Journal: A Publication of the American Academy of Osteopathy, 8*, (4), 18–21.
153. Wilberg, J. M., et al. (1999). The short-term effect of spinal manipulation in the treatment of infantile colic: A randomized controlled trial with a blinded observer. *Journal of Manipulative and Physiological Therapeutics, 22*, (8), 517–522.
154. Williams, N. H., et al. (2003). Randomized osteopathic manipulation study (ROMANS): Pragmatic trial for spinal pain in primary care. *Family Practice, 20*, (6), 662–669.
155. Zanakis, M., et al. (1993). The efficacy of OMT on spasmodic torticollis as determined by improvements in volitional movement. [Abstract.] *Journal of the American Osteopathic Association, 93*, (9), 950.
156. Zanotti, E., et al. (2012). Osteopathic manipulative treatment effectiveness in severe chronic obstructive pulmonary disease: A pilot study. *Complementary Therapies in Medicine, 20*, (1–2), 16–22.

INDEX

Page numbers followed by *f* refer to figures.

INDEX